THE ONLY CURE

Mark Solms is a leading neuropsychologist and psychoanalyst. He is the director of neuropsychology at the Neuroscience Institute of the University of Cape Town, an honorary lecturer in Neurosurgery at the St Bartholomew's & Royal London Hospital School of Medicine, and an honorary fellow of the American College of Psychiatrists. He has published widely on the brain mechanisms of dreaming, consciousness, emotion, and various neuropsychiatric disorders, and he has conducted extensive research on the integration of psychoanalytic and neuroscientific knowledge. He is the authorized editor and translator of *The Revised Standard Edition of the Complete Psychological Works of Sigmund Freud* (24 vols, 2024) and *The Complete Neuroscientific Works of Sigmund Freud* (4 vols, forthcoming). His first popular-science book, *The Hidden Spring: A Journey to the Source of Consciousness* (2021), was reviewed favourably in the *Guardian*, the *Washington Post*, *Wired* magazine, the *New Statesman* and elsewhere.

THE ONLY CURE

Freud and the Neuroscience of Mental Healing

MARK SOLMS

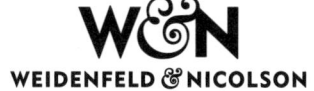

First published in Great Britain in 2026 by Weidenfeld & Nicolson,
an imprint of The Orion Publishing Group Ltd
Carmelite House, 50 Victoria Embankment
London EC4Y 0DZ

An Hachette UK Company

The authorised representative in the EEA is Hachette Ireland,
8 Castlecourt Centre, Dublin 15, D15 XTP3, Ireland (email: info@hbgi.ie)

1 3 5 7 9 10 8 6 4 2

Copyright © Mark Solms 2026

The moral right of Mark Solms to be identified as
the author of this work has been asserted in accordance
with the Copyright, Designs and Patents Act of 1988.

All rights reserved. No part of this publication may be
reproduced, stored in a retrieval system, or transmitted
in any form or by any means, electronic, mechanical,
photocopying, recording, or otherwise, without the
prior permission of both the copyright owner and the
above publisher of this book.

A CIP catalogue record for this book is
available from the British Library.

ISBN (Hardback) 978 1 3996 2337 7
ISBN (Export Trade Paperback) 978 1 3996 2338 4
ISBN (Ebook) 978 1 3996 2340 7
ISBN (Audio) 978 1 3996 2341 4

Typeset by Input Data Services Ltd, Bridgwater, Somerset
Printed in Great Britain by Elcograf, S.p.A.

www.weidenfeldandnicolson.co.uk
www.orionbooks.co.uk

In memory of my mother
ELSIE SYLVIA SOLMS, 18.6.1934–8.3.2018
with gratitude

'It may be that there are other still undreamt-of possibilities of therapy. But for the moment, we have nothing better at our disposal than the technique of psychoanalysis'

— *Sigmund Freud, 1938*

Contents

Introduction: The Symptom	1
Chapter One: Censors	15
Chapter Two: The Interpretation of Dreams	42
Chapter Three: The Mental Apparatus	64
Chapter Four: The Talking Cure	97
Chapter Five: Slips of the Tongue	129
Chapter Six: Defence Mechanisms	164
Chapter Seven: The Future of an Illusion	203
Chapter Eight: A Cure by Love	231
Epilogue: The Cause	263
Notes	277
References	289
Acknowledgements	308
Index	309

INTRODUCTION
The Symptom

To protect patient confidentiality, some details in the following story have been altered.*

But not this one: Teddy P was a doctor. By day, he worked as a trainee paediatrician in a public hospital. He was coping with the stresses of the job pretty well, until, very suddenly, his mother died. (His father had passed away while Teddy was still at medical school.)

Teddy became depressed. He started making mistakes at work. At times, he found himself unable to remember what had happened moments before. He would walk out of consultations with no memory of what he had just been talking about. What had they just agreed? His days became filled with dread, punctuated by panic attacks, overwhelming him so badly that he often had to go to the staff room to calm down.

Even before he moved in with his girlfriend, he had struggled with premature ejaculation. She was less than sympathetic about that: 'Seriously?' she exclaimed the second time it happened. Now, out of nowhere, he had erectile dysfunction to deal with as well. It seemed like a cruel joke: the damn thing would do anything but what he wanted. How was it possible that it should be simultaneously too eager and too reluctant?

After a while, his girlfriend told him she was leaving him. That wasn't a complete shock; she had already announced that she was seeing someone else. Still, he took it badly. He found it harder to sleep. Fatigue increasingly fogged his brain.

---

* Likewise for all patients described in this book.

Time to take matters in hand. Teddy did what seemed to him the natural thing: he went to a psychiatrist, who diagnosed major depressive disorder and prescribed an antidepressant. The medication helped a bit, after a month or so. Yet the sleep difficulties and the racing pulse persisted (how was it possible that his *heart* should be simultaneously too eager and too reluctant?). The psychiatrist obligingly gave him an anti-anxiety medication and a sleeping pill. Teddy developed chronic muscle pain. The psychiatrist diagnosed fibromyalgia, and wrote him a script for strong opioid painkillers.

In the months that followed, Teddy's hands began to shake. His memory got worse. His vision became blurred. Most worryingly, he was mixing up his patients, writing the wrong codes, prescribing unsuitable medications. One day he failed to recognize a girl he had examined just 24 hours earlier. Even when her mother reminded him, he had no idea who she was. Clearly, something was very seriously the matter. He asked the psychiatrist to refer him to a neurologist.

The neurologist, hearing about the blanking episodes and noticing the tremor in Teddy's hands, sent him for an EEG and a CT brain scan. The EEG revealed no epileptic activity, although it did show 'diffuse slowing'. Inconclusive. The CT showed 'mild, age-inappropriate atrophy', which is to say, general shrinkage. Again, inconclusive.

Two days later, Teddy blanked out at his home. He woke up covered in urine, with no idea how much time had passed. The neurologist ordered a second EEG. It shed no more light than the first. To be safe, he prescribed a low dose of an anti-epilepsy drug, on the basis that the absence of epileptic activity on an EEG did not rule out the possibility of seizures when doctors weren't looking. He also noted that anticonvulsants can serve as mood stabilizers, in a pinch: an additional therapeutic motivation. Belt and braces.

It was recommended that Teddy stop driving. He wasn't so far gone that he couldn't read between the lines: if he was a liability behind the wheel, he was surely a danger to his patients.

He promptly resigned from his position at the hospital and went home.

There he remained for some time.

His sleep patterns became ever more erratic – fragmented, with disturbingly vivid dreams and cold sweats. Not infrequently, he would remain in bed all day until nightfall. He stopped eating. Left alone with his thoughts, he fixated on the idea that he would never be able to return to clinical work, maybe any work, ever again.

His remaining relatives – a step-mother, an aunt, and a semi-estranged brother – reacted with alarm to this withdrawal from the world. They urged him to get a second opinion. Living, as he was, on their handouts, he had little choice but to comply. In any case, he had lost confidence in the first neurologist's vague diagnosis. He was finding it more and more difficult to concentrate, and couldn't remember what had happened from one moment to the next. Every day brought a more painful headache. His speech slurred and he struggled to find words. Names, in particular, had become almost impossible. In light of that 'mild, age-inappropriate atrophy', he was beginning to suspect that he was in fact in the first stages of some terrible degenerative disease: early-onset dementia, perhaps.

A second neurologist reviewed his EEG and CT results. She found them essentially normal, attributing the slow waves on the EEG to the multiple psychiatric medications he was taking, and the mild atrophy to normal variation. She examined him clinically and concluded that there was nothing wrong with his brain. But she could see that he was in significant distress. To be on the safe side, she referred Teddy to me.

I am a neuropsychologist. That means I specialize in the diagnosis of neurodegenerative diseases (among other things), since the indicators of most such illnesses are psychological in nature: they show up mainly as impairments in cognitive functions. I also have experience in working with 'functional' disorders: physical and cognitive conditions that appear to be neurological but are really psychiatric. Given the absence of any convincing evidence from the EEG and the scan, it seemed possible that this was what we were dealing with in this case.

I examined Teddy and reviewed his records. The pattern of his symptoms didn't remotely match any of the established neurodegenerative diseases. In any case, very few of them tend to afflict people as young as him. Alzheimer's, frontotemporal dementia, corticobasal degeneration, Lewy body disease, vascular dementia, and the like: these are diseases of the elderly, not stricken swains like the drooping young man in my office. At the same time, his symptoms seemed pretty typical of major depression and panic disorder, combined with the side effects and interactions of the many drugs he was taking. Low mood, loss of energy and appetite, problems with sleep and concentration: these were the common currency of major depression, which frequently co-occurs with panic disorder. Loss of libido (which also accompanies major depression) and vivid dreams were common side effects of SSRIs – the antidepressant drugs he was taking. Loss of memory, blurred vision and slurred speech were common with benzodiazepines – the anti-anxiety drugs he was taking. Concentration difficulties (which, again, are symptomatic of depression) are commonly compounded by anticonvulsants and hypnotics. Headaches are common with opiates; and so on.

At the end of our consultation, I told Teddy how his case seemed to me. His cognitive symptoms and motor signs were mainly *iatrogenic*: illnesses caused by the medical treatment itself. Like the old woman who swallowed a fly, most of the drugs he was taking were treating symptoms that were caused by the other drugs he was taking. Doing my best to conceal my exasperation at the treatment he had received, I said that I would recommend to his psychiatrist that she taper off almost all his medications.

Teddy was glad to hear that he didn't have dementia. Still, the prospect of stopping his drugs clearly worried him. He knew only too well how his low moods and dark thoughts could overwhelm him, how much he struggled to sleep without hypnotics, how pains would swarm his body if he couldn't have opiates. The psychiatrist was reluctant to follow my advice, too, and relented only when the neurologist strongly recommended the same.

The medications the psychiatrist had prescribed were all just *symptomatic* treatments, anyway, I told Teddy. None of them addressed the actual *causes* of his suffering. This meant that he would have to keep taking them for life. Given their side effects, and the way that the body became accustomed to some of them, meaning he would need ever higher doses to achieve the same relief, this was not advisable. The ratchet went one way only. 'But how else can I manage my symptoms?' he said. Good question.

I told him that once we had begun weaning him off his medications, he should make another appointment to see me. During that session, the focus would not be on his cognitive and other quasi-neurological symptoms, but on the story of his life. I told him I wanted to understand what had caused things to fall apart for him in the way that they had. Based on our brief acquaintance so far, I had a suspicion, but I wanted to be sure. (I didn't tell him the last part.)

Teddy gave me a strange look, as if I had done something improper, like inviting him for a drink. He thought about it.

'Alright', he said.

From this point in his story, things became more difficult. For one thing, my hunch turned out to be wide of the mark: Teddy's story was more idiosyncratic than expected. At the end of this book, I will tell you what ultimately emerged when he came to me for treatment. This isn't bait: I genuinely don't think it would make sense if I told you now. But it will.

Despite the long list of medications that my colleague prescribed for Teddy, this pharmacological tasting menu barely scrapes the surface of the range of medical specialities, hi-tech instruments and drug therapies now deployed to diagnose and treat mental suffering. Major depression alone might be treated by infusions of ketamine (a general anaesthetic), by low-dose psychedelics (like psilocybin), by vagus nerve stimulation, by ECT (electroconvulsive therapy), by TMS (transcranial magnetic stimulation), and even – albeit less frequently – by DBS (deep brain stimulation; the insertion of electrodes deep into the tissues of the brain).

All these treatments enjoy the serious stamp of science. This applies not only to the treatments and the investigations themselves, but also to the mountain of work that has gone into their development. Take the SSRI antidepressant, the first-line treatment that Teddy received. The birth of these drugs in the 1950s was followed by reams of research conducted by laboratory scientists into the variety of serotonin* receptors, the serotonin precursors and their transporters, and the genes that produce them. An equal amount of basic research has since been devoted to trying to work out what, exactly, SSRIs do. Why, for example, does it take so many weeks for them to start working, given that their primary physiological effect – increased availability of serotonin at the junctions between neurons – is immediate? All these decades later, it's amazing how little we know about them.

In 2006–12, I was research co-director of the Hope for Depression Research Foundation (HDRF), whose founder – a formidable New York billionairess whose late mother (named Hope) had suffered from severe depression – tasked me with identifying scientists around the world who were doing the most promising work, using the widest range of the latest techniques, so that she could support them. (Her ambition, it seemed to me, was not merely to advance our understanding of depression but to wipe it off the face of the earth.)

As it turned out, most of the research that the HDRF supported was conducted not upon people like Teddy P, but on laboratory rats. A particularly vexing question therefore was what a suitable 'animal model' for depression might be; that is, what the rat equivalent of depression might look like. The most widely used protocol at the time was the 'forced swim test'. The researcher

---

* The second 'S' in SSRI stands for serotonin: 'selective serotonin re-uptake inhibitors'.

placed a rat in a tank of water from which there was no escape, then measured how long it took it to stop swimming – to give up. The rats that became immobile the soonest were considered the most similar to depressed human beings. Depression, after all, is a state of hopelessness. A rat that wouldn't swim anymore was a good rat to test new treatments on.

As I got to know these leaders of depression science in the early years of the millennium, I started to feel a little downcast myself. They seemed at least as interested in the technical magic they could perform with their exciting new gadgets as they were in the prospects of actually finding a cure. Not that this research was uninteresting: much of it was very interesting, and some of it may even be valuable. All the same, it felt somehow small, and very remote from the horrible experiences of patients like Teddy P. Most depressingly, there was little prospect of these scientists actually *understanding* the disorder they were investigating. Some treatments looked a little more effective than others under experimental conditions, but the overall process was one of fumbling in the dark.

Again and again, returning to the hotel after well-funded conferences in Vienna or Cold Spring Harbor, I found myself puzzling over how little this generation of laboratory gnomes resembled the great and terrible giants who once walked the earth.

Astonishing as it seems, mainstream psychiatry was once dominated by a cadre of medical practitioners for whom *insight* was not merely the object of inquiry, but the very essence of the cure.

When I was born, 60-something years ago, it was almost impossible to obtain a tenured professorship in psychiatry at a decent American university unless you were a psychoanalyst. Psychoanalytic doctors wore flannels and tweed. Day after day, month after month, they sat listening while their patients reminisced about childhood upsets. This luxurious form of treatment occurred not in antiseptic hospital wards but in the brownstones of the Upper

East Side and the leafy avenues of Hampstead, in consulting rooms tastefully fitted in a distinctive style: chaise longue for the patient; Persian rugs on the floor if not also the walls; a scattering of Egyptian or Greco-Roman antiquities. And of course, the obligatory touch: a plaster bust or a portrait of Sigmund Freud, gazing sternly down over doctor and patient.

Psychoanalysts in those days were demigods. It wasn't just that they were widely considered to know more about what makes us tick than we could ever know ourselves (which explained why so many people would fork out such vast sums for daily consultations); the psychoanalysts themselves really did believe that they knew the hidden truths of the human condition. They saw through the muddle and happenstance of life to its core. The very workings of fate were revealed to them.

I was just a child during this heyday, but I met many of its leading lights in the 1990s, in the twilights of their careers: psychoanalytic psychiatrists such as Charles Brenner in New York, André Green in Paris, and Hannah Segal in London. I can confirm that they were not much given to self-doubt. They didn't offer opinions; they made pronouncements – even as their pedestals were crumbling beneath their feet.

In the 1960s, more than half of all American psychiatrists were psychoanalysts; today the percentage has dwindled to single figures.[1] The physicist Max Planck claimed that science progresses at the speed with which the old guard dies off. The fall of the psychoanalytic empire seemed a little quicker than that.

It was matched by the commensurately rapid rise, between the 1960s and 1980s, of what was then called 'biological psychiatry'. We don't call it that anymore. Today, almost all psychiatry is 'biological'; it is based in the certain knowledge that mental suffering is best treated *physically*, because its root causes are plainly to be found within the brain. Modern mental health practitioners and researchers are no less certain of this truth than the psychoanalysts of the past century were of theirs.

Not that this was the end of psychoanalysis. In the English-speaking world, it has survived as a form of alternative medicine, like homeopathy and acupuncture, a slightly eccentric recourse for the worried well-to-do. The situation is less dire in Latin America, Germany and France (roughly in that order), but the trend has been the same. And for the past 30 or so years, that is how it has remained.

Now, however, the ground seems to be shifting again. Since the COVID pandemic, it has become increasingly difficult to refer patients to psychoanalysts and psychoanalytic therapists (child psychotherapists, in particular) as none of them have any vacancies. Ever more psychiatrists and psychologists are applying for specialist training in psychoanalysis. Pro-Freudian opinion pieces are popping up all over the mainstream media.[2] From the depths, a figure hitherto relegated to the realm of cranks and innuendo is once again rising to the surface. Why is it happening now? What should we make of it?

Among the less controversial claims I am going to make in this book is that pretty much all modern forms of psychotherapy are derived from the work of Sigmund Freud, an Austrian neuroscientist and neurologist whose long working life took him from *fin de siècle* Vienna to Hampstead in London, where he died in exile a few weeks into the Second World War.

Many of the clichéd images of therapy derive from him: the couch, the accent, 'tell me about your mother', and so on. Freud exists now in popular imagination as a set of jokey half-remembered provocations: the Oedipus complex, penis envy, dreams reveal hidden wishes, mistakes are really intentional, sometimes a cigar is just a cigar. Even if you have never heard of these things, you'll recognize the man himself in one of his characteristic portraits: white beard, round glasses, cigar, three-piece suit. He's an icon of the intellectual culture of the previous century, like Einstein: a cartoon character.

But Freud doesn't have Einstein's saintly aura. If anything, there is something rather disreputable about him. Didn't he intimidate young women into accepting outrageous sexual interpretations of their lives? Wasn't he half crazed on cocaine? Like Karl Marx, charged with the excesses of the Soviet Union, or Friedrich Nietzsche, allegedly to blame for the atrocities of the Nazis, surely Freud must answer for much of the *nonsense* that we have to put up with: all the navel-gazing pseudoscientific know-it-all-ness that forestalled objective investigations of mental illness for a half-century or more. And while it could be argued that Marx and Nietzsche were no more responsible for Soviet and Nazi crimes than Einstein was for the nuclear arms race, Freud really was the father of therapy-speak. His ideas about trauma, or projection, or narcissism, or denial, or being 'anal', have become our folk psychology. That 'whole climate of opinion', as W. H. Auden put it,[3] that even today seems to permeate every variety of relationship, intimate, professional, and points between? That was his show.

In some ways it's surprising that his influence spread so far. Freud's account of human existence has an unsettling intimacy: childish longings, embarrassing strivings, private parts, bodily fluids, humiliating inadequacies, irretrievable losses; so many things that we would rather forget. He was always a scandalous figure, always at risk of going too far. Perhaps no theorist so discomfiting could remain in power for long. The accusations against him grew throughout the psychoanalytic century: cocaine addict, pervert, scientific fraud, bully, philanderer, patriarch, money-grabber, child-abuser, bigot, sexist, misogynist, homophobe.

The mainstream mental sciences ultimately rejected him for a variety of somewhat more sober reasons: reactions against hubris, but also intellectual fashion, and even (as we shall see) ideologies, including Stalinism. Yet in a peculiar way, psychoanalysis also rejected Freud. The field today tends not to be interested in, or even to recognize, his deep aspirations as a scientist. Freud's theories were always meant to answer to the evidence, even when it was obtained from other fields of inquiry; and his psychological model was always waiting to make firm contact with brain research once again. The prophet of today's psychoanalysts, and the disreputable old man of popular stereotype, are much less interesting, much less challenging figures, than the dedicated and serious scientist that I have come to know over the course of my career. That is the Freud I would like to introduce you to now.

Among the more controversial claims that I am going to defend in this book is that we need him today more than ever.

I have been a neuroscientist all my working life. I started investigating the brain mechanisms of sleep and dreaming in 1985, before extending my research to take in the anatomy and physiology of consciousness in general, and the close relationship between sentience and emotion. Along the way, I studied the brain mechanisms of psychiatric conditions such as major depression, panic disorder and addiction, and of neurobehavioural disorders such as Korsakoff syndrome (confabulatory amnesia) and anosognosia (unawareness of being paralysed). From this work, I have published more than 300 peer-reviewed scientific journal articles and book chapters, and I have authored several technical books.

Unlike many neuroscientists, I am also a clinician. I have treated all the conditions just mentioned – both the psychiatric and the neurological ones – and participated in neurosurgical treatments of other conditions, such as brain tumours, pharmacologically intractable epilepsy and Parkinson's disease.

More unusually, I decided in the late 1980s to train as a psychoanalyst – much to the dismay of my neuroscientific colleagues. I have practised psychotherapy and psychoanalysis for many years. This apparently eccentric sideline led me to engage deeply with Freud's writings, to the extent of producing scholarly editions of much of his published and unpublished output – including English translations of his early neuroscientific and neurological papers, and those of some other 19th-century neurologists.

This gives me a rare, although not a unique, vantage point on the development of mental science over the past century, and especially on changes that took place during the last four decades. Among the most surprising patterns that I have observed is this.

From the 1970s onwards, just when mental science was officially turning away from psychoanalysis, fragmentary evidence from all manner of experimental studies in many different fields began to coalesce into a big picture that we might call the modern scientific model of the mind. It is, not to beat about the bush, astonishingly like the one Freud sketched out in the first decades of the 20th century. Much as it might suit the pride of neuroscience to call this a coincidence, it is not. It is a testament to genuinely deep insights, attributable to Freud and then fruitfully developed by some of his followers, into how the mind really works.

This is of course *interesting*, in an abstract way, as a piece of intellectual history. But it's more than that, too. My conviction, formed both in the trenches of mental healthcare and in a long research career, is that this convergence of modern neuroscience and the half-forgotten conjectures of psychoanalysis is actually important. As I will argue, Freud gleaned his remarkable insights precisely because of the angle from which he examined the mind. He looked, not from the perspective of brain anatomy and physiology, but from the vantage point of *being* a mind. Freud (and with varying levels of rigour, his followers) undertook to map the organization of the mind as it manifests *subjectively*.

Neuroscience has to an impressive degree refused to avail itself of this perspective. There are semi-good reasons for this – not least that science aims for objectivity. Yet it is surely a fundamental feature of the brain, seemingly alone among all the organs of the body and every other object in the known universe, that it does possess a subjective perspective; that there is, as philosophers say, 'something it is like' to be one.[4]

This extraordinary attribute must have evolved for a reason. That in turn implies that it must make a difference to how the brain works. Is it not obviously true that what you *feel* influences what you *do*? Denying this is tantamount to excluding the psyche from psychology.

Freud's view was that we must adjust our methods of observation to our objects of study, not the other way around. Accordingly, he and his followers achieved many novel insights into the nature and organization of the mind that are only now being rediscovered by neuroscience. They cover everything from the meaning of suffering to the structure of memory to the significance of childhood. I will describe nine of them in the chapters that follow. It's a great shame that ideological opposition to Freud in the later 20th century has held neuroscience up for so long.

If that's a shame, what it has meant for mental healthcare is nothing less than a scandal. Let me say it bluntly, here at the outset: nearly every psychiatric disorder listed and defined in the standard diagnostic manuals is best understood and treated, not pharmacologically, but psychologically. This applies even to some mental conditions originating in genetic predispositions and in physical brain disease. As things stand, physiological treatments of psychiatric disorders are limited to the temporary relief of symptoms, and psychiatric understanding is close to being a contradiction in terms. Not that relief of symptoms cannot be valuable at times, to pave the way to more enduring causal treatments. But there are, as things stand, no physiological cures in psychiatry.

And yet, for many disorders, a causal treatment has been available all along.

As we shall see, there is now a mountain of evidence that the mainstream psychotherapies derived from psychoanalysis are astoundingly effective. That goes even more so for psychoanalysis itself – not only when compared to other psychiatric interventions such as the drugs prescribed for Teddy P, but also when compared to regular medical treatments for common physical ailments. Even relatively brief courses of psychoanalysis deserve to be described as 'highly effective' by the standard medical definition of that term, and not by a narrow margin. For certain conditions, they are as dependable as, say, insulin is at managing type 1 diabetes, or as the HPV vaccine is at preventing cervical cancer. These treatments are so well proven that it would strike most doctors as – to use a technical term – crazy not to deploy them by default.

Why does psychoanalysis work so well? And why do patients treated on Freudian lines reliably *continue to get better long after treatment has ceased*? This isn't 'regression to the mean', or people naturally getting better over time. It's a very distinctive effect of the therapies derived from Freud's ideas. It is most strongly visible in the treatments that hew closest to his original methods. As I hope to convince you, the reason for the pattern is this: psychoanalysis actually gets to the root of the problem. The talking cure is a cure – and still the only real one we have in psychiatry.

This is not a self-help book. For the really difficult, really deep problems, you actually can't fix them by yourself, whatever some authors might suggest. If I explain a bit of what is ultimately going on in various types of mental disorder, that won't put me and my colleagues out of work. Even so, I hope to give readers who have no professional stake in these subjects a rough-and-ready map to the mind that is not just interesting but also *useful*. It can be consoling to view one's problems in the light of what has been learnt from treating similar problems in thousands of other people. And it can illuminate one's existence in countless big and small ways to have a general sense of how the mental apparatus as a whole fits together.

That's what I offer in the pages that follow: the core insights of psychoanalysis, clarified and updated with the best of modern neuroscience. Together they yield a single, intuitive scheme that explains in broad terms what is going on inside the heads of each one of us, in sickness and in health, in sleep and waking, in our public lives and the deepest privacy of our souls, which in the end no censor can quiet.

'Our science', wrote Freud in 1927, 'is no illusion. But an illusion it would be to suppose that what science cannot give us we can get elsewhere.'[5]

CHAPTER ONE
Censors

ANALYST: It wasn't meant to be a statement of fact. It was meant to be a kind of 'Is this what you're feeling?', for you to say yes or no. I was asking: talking to an authority, does it make you feel boxed in?
PATIENT: But I said no, it doesn't, and you still carried on. I will never agree with you making me out to be a paranoid person. I am not that way.
ANALYST: What makes you say paranoid?
PATIENT: Because of authority; your focus on authority, my relationship with authority. Most people who have paranoid personalities have problems with authority.
ANALYST: They think everybody's trying to harm them. Not just authority figures.
PATIENT: It starts with authority figures. I've known a few schizophrenics. It always starts with the government; it never starts with the common person.

— From the author's clinical files

The ancient Egyptians didn't think much of the brain. When preparing a body for the afterlife, they scooped it out via the nose and threw it away. Ancient Chinese doctors similarly deemed it of little importance; it was the heart that determined our individual qualities and the understanding of sensory perceptions. The Greek philosopher Aristotle agreed, seeing the heart as the seat of our sentient being. The comparatively lowly task he assigned to the brain was to cool the body down.

It seems to have been Hippocrates who turned the tide, around 400 BCE. As a physician, he conducted many autopsies, and perhaps it was this experience that revealed to him how many patients with mental abnormalities in life turn out on the dissection table to have damaged or diseased brains. Galen, another ancient Greek doctor, developed the insight and observed that the mysterious organ in the skull was connected with the rest of the body by a network of nerves, which he thought were tubes. Interestingly, he believed it was the hollow sacs or ventricles within the brain that contained the soul, rather than the actual tissues. Presumably this emphasis on the circulatory systems – initially on the flow of blood through the body and then on the transparent fluid that circulates through the tubes and ventricles – reflected the *immaterial* nature of the soul. Building upon a belief passed down to him by more-ancient ancients to the effect that 'animal spirits' contain the elements, earth, air, fire and water, Galen proposed that four 'humours' circulate through the body – black bile, blood, yellow bile and phlegm – and he claimed that imbalances in these make you melancholic, sanguine, choleric and phlegmatic, respectively.

This remained the state of the art in brain anatomy for about 14 centuries. At the dawn of the Enlightenment, the mathematician René Descartes declared the tiny pineal gland to be the seat of the soul, apparently on the basis of its central location, floating just behind the ventricles. Under the influence of Thomas Willis, British empiricists like Locke and Hume finally focused upon the matter of the brain itself, concluding that vibrations, rather than fluids, are transmitted along the nerves connecting it with the sense organs, leaving impressions – memory images – in its cortical cells, one image per cell. These impressions then became associated with each other by way of the connections between the cells to form ideas. The phrenologists Gall and Spurzheim fancied that the ideas, in turn, grouped together to form various mental 'faculties', whose relative significance could be determined by examining the bumps on each person's cranium: the bigger the bump, the more developed the faculty. One of these faculties, language, was attributed to the frontal lobes of the brain; and that attribution happened (by chance) to be correct, more or less.

In 1861, Paul Broca reported to an astonished audience that the capacity for language was abolished in a patient named Monsieur Leborgne, who was found at autopsy to have localized damage in the third left frontal convolution of his brain. In the next four years, Broca found 12 more cases with the same mental deficit associated with the same frontal brain lesion. 'There are in the human mind a group of faculties and in the brain groups of convolutions', he wrote, 'and the facts assembled by science so far allow us to state [. . .] that the great regions of the mind correspond to the great regions of the brain.'[1] With that, neuropsychology was born.

The human brain, we are constantly told, is the most complicated object in the known universe. A hundred billion neurons, a hundred trillion synaptic connections – more connections than stars in the Milky Way. 'If the brain were so simple that we could understand it,' I once saw scratched on a toilet cubicle door in a British medical school, 'we would be so simple that we couldn't.' That may be, but we still have to live with it, as we do the climate, the stock market, politics, and many things of almost overwhelming complexity. It's too important to ignore. So, we do the best we can.

Over the centuries, there have been many attempts to get to grips with the problem, to simplify it and make it tractable. The investigators differed in their modes of investigation, in their theoretical presuppositions, and in the kinds of data they took to be significant. Some of them were decidedly far-fetched. Astrology had a spectacular run as our leading science of human personality, crystallizing in the Hellenistic world around 300 BCE and showing no sign of vanishing from the popular imagination just yet. The bumps on your head are arguably more credible determinants of your personal qualities than the stars in the sky, but despite its early success, phrenology also slipped out of the running as a serious scientific programme, relegated to a dustier section of the occult shop even than astrology and Tarot (and, for that matter, certain books of psychoanalytic theory).

All these accounts of the soul – inspired, insane, prosaic or profane – jostled against one another in uneasy coexistence. It would take a very open mind to suggest that they each possess a part of the truth. Yet, whatever their differences, they are all vantage points upon, and attempts to explain, the same thing, namely what we *are*: How does the mind work? And how does it relate to our bodies?

Progress came, as it often does, in the form of agreement. Over time, some of these nascent sciences started to corroborate one another, and finally they settled on a basic story.

Here it is, in a nutshell.

The soul (renamed the mind) derives from sensory experience, in the form of *memories*. These are stored in different zones of the cortex that receive information from the senses, and they are associated with one another to form the various mental faculties (renamed *functions*).

It might not sound like much, but it was a start.

After Broca's localization of language, reports emerged, first in Europe and then all over the world, of innumerable other cases in which deficits in various mental functions followed damage to other specific parts of the cortex. The race to localize these functions in various brain 'centres' (as they were called) resulted in an impressively comprehensive map.[2] Yet it lacked precision. Neurologists couldn't help but notice that damage to the different centres didn't produce deficits in just the one mental function assigned to it; and even when it did, the function wasn't lost completely. Thus, for example, patients with damage in what has come to be known as 'Broca's area' were still capable of producing concrete words like nouns, but they lost the connecting ones. A patient with Broca's aphasia who wants to say 'could you please pass me the salt' might say, haltingly, 'you . . . me . . . salt'. Rather than total loss of language, their speech is characterized by what is called 'agrammatism'. So, we have a mystery. Is language stored in Broca's area, or isn't it?

The Canadian psychologist Donald Hebb coined the word 'neuropsychology' in 1949, and many others contributed to the early development of the field,* but nobody is more deserving of the epithet 'father of neuropsychology' than a brilliant Russian neurologist named Aleksandr Romanovich Luria (1902–77).

Luria's inspired answer to the puzzle of Broca's area, and the more general question of why mental functions do not map directly onto cortical centres, was this: they are *distributed*. Mental functions like language, Luria argued, are akin to bodily processes such as respiration or digestion. Such complex functions cannot be localized narrowly in the tissues of the lungs or the stomach. Respiration entails the expansion of the intercostal muscles of the diaphragm, which draws air through the trachea, which oxygenates the blood in the alveoli of the lungs, which is pumped to other organs by the heart, and so on. The functions of each of these tissues may be described as 'components' of the system as a whole, but the total function is not performed *in* any one of them. What matters is the interaction *between* them.

This dynamically distributed nature of mental functions seemed particularly promising when it came to the second puzzle about Broca-style localizationism. How did the transmission of nerve impulses from cells in the sense organs to cells in the cerebral cortex turn into *ideas*? Or, to put it another way, how does a purely physiological process become a subjective experience?

Luria's response to this one was subtle. He said that the mental symptoms arising from brain injuries must be analysed in their

---

* Such as the American neurologist Norman Geschwind, the French psychiatrist Henry Hécaen, the German-American psychologist Hans-Lukas Teuber, the British psychologist Oliver Zangwill, and the American neurosurgeon Karl Pribram.

own right, psychologically, and *functionally*, not physiologically. This turned out to be a fateful distinction. When we investigate the function of some organ or system, we ask what it does, saving for another day the more concrete question of exactly how it does it. When we investigate the physiology of an organ or system, by contrast, we try to understand immediately how its bodily tissues perform the function in question – like the alveoli of the lungs in relation to respiration. Means and ends: physiology provides the means to a functional end.

For Luria, accordingly, neuropsychological science did not entail *reduction* of complex psychological functions to simple physiological mechanisms, but rather what he called 'qualification'. He was interested in the peculiar psychological character of each mental impairment, and the pattern of other psychological symptoms that occurred alongside it. The thing you could describe in physiological terms – the thing that could be assigned to specific anatomical tissues – was not the mental capacity as a whole, but just a component, which might play a part in many different functions.* To map entire psychological systems, such as those for language or memory, you had to note *all* the deficits arising from each little piece of tissue damage. 'The singling out of a symptom is not the end but rather the beginning of [this] work, which continues in depth,' Luria wrote.[3] Only when he had the full clinical picture could he begin to look for an underlying factor that might explain each of the psychological observations. He called this process 'dynamic localization'.

Like the other pioneers of neuropsychology, Luria developed his major insights in the wake of the Second World War. In 1943, he took charge of an 800-bed military hospital for patients with traumatic brain injuries. This was fortunate (for him), since the method of dynamic localization required the detailed examination of multiple injuries at different locations throughout the brain's

---

* The same components participate in multiple functional systems; so neuropsychological syndromes frequently involve impairments in several different mental faculties simultaneously.

entire anatomy. The Soviet military's astonishingly high casualty rate during the war furnished him with plenty of raw data, and Luria set out some of his resulting insights in a monograph titled *Traumatic Aphasia* (1947), in which he reconceptualized Broca's and the other aphasias in the terms described above. Almost immediately, it brought him to world renown.

From the 1950s onwards, at leading international conferences of neurologists and psychologists, Luria was a star speaker. In the following three decades, he published *Restoration of Functions after Brain Injury* (1948), *Human Brain and Psychological Processes* (1963), *The Psychophysiology of the Frontal Lobes* (1973, with Karl Pribram), *Basic Problems of Neurolinguistics* (1975), *The Neuropsychology of Memory* (1976) – and his two most famous case studies, *The Mind of a Mnemonist* (1968) and *The Man with a Shattered World* (1972).

His greatest work, however, was undoubtedly the magisterial *Higher Cortical Functions in Man* (1962), whose essential findings he summarized in more digestible form in another celebrated book, *The Working Brain* (1973). These two volumes were the main textbooks we studied when I trained in neuropsychology in the early 1980s.* Like many neuropsychological colleagues around the world, I have used Luria's method of investigation in my four decades of clinical practice, to diagnose and treat innumerable kinds of brain disease and brain injury in thousands of patients. I, together with my colleagues and our patients, owe an immense debt to his foundational work. The validity of his most basic insight – namely, that mental life arises from interactions between multiple component functions located in widely distributed parts of the brain – is taken for granted now; so much so, in fact, that nobody bothers to ask where it came from.

---

* We used *Higher Cortical Function in Man* in its second (1980) English-language edition.

Many neuroscientists are taken aback to learn that Luria began his scientific career as a psychoanalyst. (Some of them might find it more acceptable if he had got his start studying witchcraft.) And yet, it's true. Shortly after graduating in 1921 with a degree in biology and social science, Luria founded a psychoanalytical society in his hometown of Kazan. He wrote to Freud in 1922 to inform him, and there followed a brief correspondence in which Freud recognized the new society and addressed Luria as 'Herr President'. One suspects he didn't realize he was writing to a teenager.[4]

During the seventeen scientific meetings that the Kazan Psychoanalytic Association held between September 1922 and September 1923, Luria delivered twelve lectures on a wide range of psychoanalytical topics. These included 'Some Principles of Psychoanalysis', 'Psychoanalysis in Light of the Main Tendencies in Modern Psychology', 'The Current Crisis in Russian Psychology' and 'The Present State of Psychoanalysis'. He also reported the results of his empirical research, such as a study on sleep-onset fantasies, and he analysed patients at the Kazan Psychiatric Hospital (including, incidentally, Fyodor Dostoevsky's granddaughter).[5]

In late 1923, Luria moved to Moscow, where he undertook postgraduate studies in linguistics and – later – completed his medical training. There he joined the Russian Psychoanalytical Society and became its secretary. This society was extremely active: it included not only a scientific and educational programme but also a publishing house, an outpatient clinic, and a kindergarten for troubled children.

Over the next five years, Luria continued to pursue his intensive programme of psychoanalytical research, and he continued to write about diverse psychoanalytic topics. In 1925, for example, he wrote an introduction (with Lev Vygotsky) to the Russian translation of one of Freud's most important books, *Beyond the Pleasure Principle* (1920). His ongoing research included a series of studies on dreams in which he suggested 'latent' dream thoughts to people under hypnosis and observed how these were transformed into the 'manifest' content of dreams. Freud had inferred unconscious (latent) wishes from consciously remembered (manifest) dreams, retrospectively; Luria wanted to test the theory by implanting the unconscious wishes in advance.

On March 17, 1927, Luria presented a discussion of a recently published book by Bernard Bykhovsky, titled *Freud's Metapsychology* (1926). The book's main argument was that the psychoanalytic account of the drives that underpin human psychology was compatible with Marxism-Leninism. Luria agreed that it was. Three weeks later, however, seemingly without warning, he asked to be relieved of his duties as secretary of the Society. He made no further contributions to its scientific and other activities, and within two years he resigned from it altogether.

After this, Luria didn't have much more to say about psychoanalysis, or not in public, anyway. Ten years later, in 1940, he was asked to write an entry on the subject for *The Great Soviet Encyclopaedia*. He must have accepted this dubious honour nervously. In his entry, he dismissed psychoanalysis as a 'false theory' belonging to 'the sphere of hostile advanced science', on the grounds that it 'biologizes the complex, historically-determined conscious state of the human being'.[6]

He never discussed Freudian theory in his published writings again, apart from a brief mention in his autobiography, in which he repented his youthful dalliance:

> Here, I thought, was a scientific approach that combined a strongly deterministic explanation of concrete, individual behaviour with an explanation of the origins of complex human needs in terms of natural science. Perhaps psychoanalysis could serve as the basis for a scientific *reale Psychologie*, one that would overcome the nomothetic-ideographic distinction [. . .] But I finally concluded that it was an error to assume that one can deduce human behaviour from the biological 'depths' of the mind, excluding its social 'heights'.[7]

This is a surprising line for him to have taken, given that the remainder of his career concerned nothing but the biological 'depths' of the mind. As a neuropsychologist, Luria investigated mental phenomena in their most general and fundamental – it is tempting to say elemental – forms, right down to their physiological and anatomical roots.

In *The Working Brain* (1973), which was written shortly before his death in 1977, Luria summarized his life's work under the following chapter headings: 'Perception', 'Movement and Action', 'Attention', 'Memory', 'Language' and 'Thinking'. In the concluding chapter, he wrote the following:

> Neuropsychology is still a very young science, taking its very first step, and a period of thirty years is not a very long time for the development of any science. That is why some very important chapters, such as motives, complex forms of emotions and the structure of personality are not included in this book. Perhaps they will be added in future editions.[8]

Alas, not by him. For those unschooled in the wisdom of giving certain subjects a wide berth, the three missing chapters may seem like a puzzling lacuna. Surely motives, emotions and the structure of personality are fundamental aspects of the mind! In Western neuroscience, there was a standard story as to why you should avoid these topics, and we will examine it in a moment. For now, let's just note that this standard explanation was not the one that Luria gave when he recanted his earlier enthusiasm for psychoanalysis, and it almost certainly wasn't what dissuaded him.

The real reason for Luria's sudden change of heart is not difficult to guess. Many historians of the period[9] have documented how, as Stalin strengthened his grip on the Communist Party between 1924 and 1929, attacks on psychoanalysis began to appear in the Soviet press. This included direct personal denunciations of Luria himself, who was accused of 'essentialism' and even colonialism. (Essentialism is the idea that we have natural characteristics that are inherent and unchanging.) By 1930 – the year in which he resigned from the Russian Psychoanalytical Society – 'psychoanalysis became a *scientia non grata* in the Soviet Union'.[10] Many of Luria's former colleagues were blacklisted, some were executed, and 'those who survived lived in an atmosphere of total suspicion'.[11] After he was denounced and 'found guilty of ideological deviations',[12] his resignation and subsequent public disavowals of his previous views were 'the only way he would be able to continue his important work'.[13]

Why exactly did the Soviet Union turn against psychoanalysis? An interesting question. Opinions among senior party authorities in the immediate wake of the 1917 revolution differed regarding the compatibility of Freudian theory with Marxist doctrine: Trotsky, for example, shared Luria's admiration for Bykhovsky's bridge-building book, *Freud's Metapsychology*; Stalin decidedly did not. By 1930, however, differing opinions had become dangerous. Trotsky was in exile (eventually to be assassinated) and orthodoxy reigned. The new orthodoxy was Stalin's.

The Stalinist case against Freud is difficult to reconstruct, in part because it wasn't rational. The accusation that psychoanalysis 'biologized' the mind boiled down to the view that mental conflict isn't something that exists within the individual but rather between social classes: between organized labour and capital. Freud considered that our conflicted nature is rooted in fundamentally incompatible biological urges, and in the inherent tension between all these inner needs on the one hand and the constraints of outer reality (including society) on the other. In short, he found conflict to be an unavoidable fact of life. This did not sit well with the view that an historic victory by labour over capital would shortly culminate in a communist utopia.

More troubling for Stalin personally, perhaps, was the claim that the social constraints imposed on our pleasure-seeking drives included those laid down during childhood by parental authority figures, which were internalized in the form of a mental agency that Freud called the 'superego'. In the symbolic struggle between libertarian children and authoritarian parents, it is easy to see which side Stalin would be on. It is equally clear which side he would have associated with the troublesome Leon Trotsky. Trotsky believed that psychoanalysis (which seeks to undo psychological repression) was compatible with Marxism (which seeks to undo socioeconomic repression).

There was a further, still more personal complication. Trotsky supported, both politically and financially, the Russian Psychoanalytical Society's foundation in 1926 of its kindergarten in Moscow. It so happens that among the school's first intake was Stalin's youngest son, Vasily, then aged five. Vasily grew into a very troubled man and died of chronic alcoholism. Stalin's antipathy to psychoanalysis probably can't be reduced entirely to personal grudges, but he was hardly an enlightened intellectual. He was petty, authoritarian and ruthless, and after Lenin's death in 1924, Trotsky was his most serious rival for control of the party.

At the very least, it seems safe to say that Trotsky's enthusiasm for psychoanalysis would not have helped its cause in Soviet Russia. As the educationalist Yordanka Valkanova wrote: 'Trotsky's involvement was also unfortunate and provoked adverse actions. Soon after Stalin launched a series of attacks on Trotsky in 1924, the [psychoanalytic] project was labelled "anti-Marxist".'[14]

And did I mention that Stalin was deeply antisemitic, and that Freud (like Trotsky and Luria) was a Jew?

These are all persuasive considerations in their ways, especially since no way other than Stalin's was permitted. Yet they aren't scientific arguments. Accordingly, Luria's sudden abandonment of psychoanalysis was unlikely to have been motivated by scientific considerations. As many historians of the period have pointed out, and as many of his friends and colleagues have told me, the change in his scientific direction was only a change of research methods. His private theoretical views remained unchanged.

Alex Kozulin, the Russian educationalist and author of *Psychology in Utopia* (1984), writes: 'Published papers and official records must be taken not at face value but rather as rough material for subsequent distillation and decoding.'¹⁵ He adds: 'In the case of Luria, it is not quite clear whether his renunciation of psychoanalysis in the 1930s was a result of, or a form of resistance against, the silencing of the topic.'¹⁶

The historian of Soviet science, David Joravsky, writes:

> Luria always managed to maintain professional integrity within his discipline, while adapting himself to the requirements of the authorities without. The subtle combination of inner autonomy and outward compliance has been a characteristic feature [. . .] in Luria's response to [. . .] Stalinism.¹⁷

Luria's biographer, Michael Cole, writes:

> When I correlated the content and style of his writings with the general political and social controversies of the day, the otherwise disjointed, zigzag course of Alexander Romanovich's career began to make sense. His interest in psychoanalysis no longer appeared a curious anomaly [. . .] His apparent shifts of topic at frequent intervals, all took on the quality of an intricate piece of music with a few central motifs and a variety of secondary themes.¹⁸

It is significant that, although from 1928 the word 'psychoanalysis' no longer appeared in Luria's publications (experimental studies of free association, for example, and clinical studies of the development of mental functions in normal and abnormal children),* his ongoing work kept being cited in Grinstein's (1956–75) *Index of*

---

* Other work by Luria in the immediate post-psychoanalytic period included a field-study of cultural differences in thinking, conducted with a group of colleagues, in which Luria concentrated on 'visual thinking' (as he had done in his research on dreams and fantasies) and 'self-analysis and evaluation of other individuals at various stages of personality development' (Luria, 1932b, p. 242). See also Luria & Vygotsky's intriguing book on *Ape, Primitive Man and Child* (1930), which appeared in English translation in 1992.

Psychoanalytic Writings right up to 1968. The continuity is perhaps most obvious in Luria's book on *The Nature of Human Conflicts* (1932a). This monograph – which described (and measured) the effects upon behaviour of emotional conflicts, and release from such conflicts – was based directly upon the research that he initiated while he was a member of the Russian Psychoanalytical Society. He scrupulously avoided both the name of Freud and the language of psychoanalysis in its pages.

The neurologist Oliver Sacks, who was a friend of Luria's, believed that the key to his enthusiasm for psychoanalysis was the way it bridged the objective and subjective perspectives. In fact, this is exactly what Luria admitted in his autobiography (quoted above). Sacks added that he never really lost that enthusiasm. In a 1985 letter to me, for example, Sacks recalled:

> In December '75 I sent him [Luria] a tape of (the verbal and vocal tics of) a patient of mine with severe Tourette's syndrome. Among these, but ejaculated with such speed as to seem at first a meaningless noise, was the word *'Verboten!'* ['forbidden!'], uttered in a harsh (indeed parodied) 'Teutonic' voice, and at times (and in a manner suggestive of) self-recrimination. This had, it later turned out, been spat out by the patient's German-speaking father whenever his son showed 'impermissible' tics and impulses. The confirmation of this, indeed the following up of it, was initiated by Luria's letter [in response to the tape], in early '76, when he suggested that I study '. . . the introjection of father as tic' . . . Luria said, or felt able to say, in letters a good deal that he felt (externally or internally) unable to say in print – and this made me feel that he was still, at least, sympathetic to psychoanalysis as a tool and dynamic description of value.[19]

In the 1976 letter to Sacks, Luria referred also to 'the structuralization of super-ego'. This is an undisguisably psychoanalytic formulation, referring to the Stalinist part of the mind mentioned earlier: the voice of the internalized, punitive father.

The psychologist Luciano Mecacci, who worked with Luria in the 1970s, writes that '[Luria's] clinical approach to the study of neuropsychological disorders undoubtedly sprang from his early experiences in psychoanalysis in the 1920s'. He continues:

> As anyone who saw Luria at work at the Burdenko Institute of Neurosurgery in Moscow would have noted, his approach to patients was purely clinical, closer to the psychoanalytic style than that of the experimentalistic attitude towards behaviour. He had no fixed schedule for interviewing and testing a patient, but he employed a free association technique, selecting the questions and the test trials according to what emerged in the session. Finally, this mode of neuropsychological investigation was unique with each patient, and might not be replicated with another patient [. . .] The neuropsychological 'portrait' that emerged from this clinical investigation fit[ted] in with the conception of the historical character of an individual's psychological life.[20]

The theoretical framework that Luria adopted explicitly in *The Nature of Human Conflicts*, after his public renunciation of psychoanalysis, was that of the English neurologist John Hughlings Jackson. There is an exquisite irony in the fact that this is precisely the framework that Freud adopted in 1891, in one of his last neurological publications, on the subject of aphasia – the very topic that Luria turned his attention to after he supposedly abandoned Freudian theory. The neuropsychology of language was a safe subject in Stalin's Russia, as were all the other topics that Luria listed as chapter headings in his 1973 summary of his life's work, because they concerned *cognition* rather than the far trickier and more interesting topics that he had researched before the 1930s: human motivation, emotion, and the structure of personality.

I suggest that, for very good reasons, Luria retreated from the most dangerous frontiers of his research and disavowed the origin of the intellectual framework in which it ultimately made sense. To escape the sanction of the censor, he maimed and disguised his project. In its inner logic, however, it remained essentially Freudian.

This rather mutilated version of neuropsychology was the version that I inherited when I entered the field in the 1980s. For the avoidance of doubt, I am not suggesting that neuropsychologists in the West gave Freud a wide berth because they were afraid of Stalin, or were obtusely following in the footsteps of a man who was. Neither would I wish to characterize objections to psychoanalysis as essentially Stalinist in any extended, pejorative sense. The story I have told of A. R. Luria is simply true as far as it concerns itself; and insofar as it concerns the later development of his field, it offers at most a suggestive allegory.

Yet there really was a wider chill in the mental sciences from the 1960s onward. Though it happened later, and to a much less deadly degree, psychoanalysis became a *scientia non grata* in the West, too. We might characterize the general attitude that I encountered in the 1980s as one of *reticence*: a sudden, collective, socially reinforced aversion. It looked, in other words, like a reaction. As I hope to show, the severity of this reaction far exceeded the warrant of its rational motivations.

At times, in psychoanalytic writing, it can be difficult to tell whether you are reading science or literature. Freud himself wrote in his *Studies on Hysteria* (1895):

> It still strikes me myself as strange that the case histories I write should read like short stories and that, as one might say, they lack the serious stamp of science. I must console myself with the reflection that the nature of the subject is evidently responsible for this, rather than any preference of my own.[21]

The direct cause of Freud's eventual dethronement in the West was not the fact that he published case histories of individual patients; these are commonplace in neurology and in medicine generally. The problem was that Freud's case histories conveyed the *subjective* perspective of the patient. Subjectivity has always been the avowed enemy of science, since Galileo. Yet Freud's topic was 'the nature of the subject'. How else could he proceed but by taking his patients' own experience seriously?

To make matters worse, he wanted to know what *lay behind* subjective experience. He was interested not only in what we can transparently learn about ourselves by looking inward, but also what remains hidden. This, of course, involves a degree of conjecture: the psychoanalyst considers all the available facts and then infers the most likely explanation. And by the second half of the 20th century, this innocent-sounding procedure had come under a new kind of suspicion.

In his great work, *Conjectures and Refutations* (1963), the philosopher Karl Popper addressed the question of how scientific knowledge is achieved. Given his immense and lasting stature among scientific practitioners (every natural scientist I know subscribes to his philosophy), it is perhaps surprising that Popper decided that scientific knowledge could never be achieved. He declared that a scientific theory can only be proven false; it can never be verified. After all, he observed, for any finite set of empirical observations, there are many possible hypotheses that might fit them. What if the most obvious pattern is not the true one? You can keep adding new data and ruling out rival conjectures as long as you want, but no amount of research is sufficient to rule out *all* possible rival hypotheses. No matter how broad or exacting your examination, the rules and mechanisms that really determine what happens might not be what you think they are. At best, provided we aren't contradicted by the evidence, we are permitted only to *hope* that our theories are getting *closer* to the truth.

> This procedure has no natural end. Thus if the test is to lead us anywhere, nothing remains but to stop at some point or other and say that we are satisfied, for the time being.[22]

How disappointing. Yet Popper's logic does allow us to know one very useful thing. We can know when our theories are *wrong*. When we make a conjecture about the workings of whatever part of nature interests us, and deduce a prediction from that conjecture, the failure of the prediction lets us know that the conjecture must be mistaken in some way. Good news! We have learned something. For Popper (and his followers; that is, for the mainstream of Western philosophy of science) the mark of a properly scientific theory is that it generates predictions that can in principle be tested and found wanting in this way. Such a theory is 'falsifiable': it asserts something, rather in the way that a bet asserts something.

What, then, of theories that entail no definite predictions about what we should expect to observe in an experimental test of them? Theories that can't be so tested are, to borrow a phrase from the physicist Wolfgang Pauli, 'not even wrong'.[23] (If their proponents don't seem sufficiently interested in falsification, they might even meet the criterion suggested by the philosopher Harry Frankfurt: 'It is just this lack of connection to a concern with truth – this indifference to how things really are – that I regard as the essence of bullshit.')[24]

Theories that have been falsified are not scientific, but theories that could not be put to the test of falsification are something much worse: they are pseudoscience – like Galen's humoral theory, or like any other incoherent bid to decipher the workings of the universe. And that might not always be an innocent mistake: to knowingly clothe oneself in the authority of science without paying the dues is a form of charlatanry. Since 1963, then, a verdict of pseudoscience has been the death-knell for any scientific theory.

Viewed from the Popperian perspective, psychoanalysis was always on thin ice. Its data points were the thoughts and feelings of individual persons. Such data arise only within the privacy of their individual minds, placing them beyond the reach of objective research. Solo introspection, the only alternative, is muddled or imperfect, even while we keep our gaze trained inwards, and it is further distorted in the memory thereafter; and first-person testimony, which, in addition to these faults, can also be deceptive (either deliberately or unwittingly, or somewhere in between) and misunderstood, especially given the prevalence of linguistic ambiguity where subjective matters are at stake. What is more, psychoanalysis tasks itself with accounting for precisely these apparent defects: the muddle, the lapses of memory, the deceptions witting and unwitting, the prevalence of ambiguity – the motive forces, in short, *behind* all the confused appearances of our private inner worlds.

Actually, it's even worse than that. The centrepiece of Freudian theory rests upon perhaps the flimsiest type of data ever adduced in a scientific context: dream reports. *Dream reports!* Retrospective, subjective first-person descriptions of notoriously confusing hallucinatory episodes that occur during sleep, and which are proverbial for being hard to remember. Not content with snatching these wisps from the void, the psychoanalyst further insists that they don't even mean what they appear to mean. According to Freud's classical doctrine, dreams are strangely wilful obfuscations and contradictions of their own underlying subject matter, which is always a desire too disturbing to show its face in the daylight of conscious reflection. Thus, psychoanalysis proceeds by gathering 'free associations' to the given details of each dream, until they seem to divulge a pattern: the secret wish that the patient's consciousness had sought (in the jargon) to repress.

How could the results of such a procedure ever be falsified? Clearly, there is nothing to stop an analyst 'interpreting' any patient's dream in such a way as to reveal an unconscious wish. Neither the patient nor anyone else can prove the negative, not even in the case of nightmares. (Freud's explanation of nightmares was that they are *failed* attempts to fulfil repressed wishes.) Popper invited the reader to imagine two contrasting situations: that of a man who pushes a child into the water with the intention of drowning it, and that of a man who drowns in an attempt to save the child.

> According to Freud the first man suffered from repression (say, of some component of his Oedipus complex), while the second man had achieved sublimation [. . .] I could not think of any human behaviour which could not be interpreted in terms of either theory. It was precisely this fact – that they always fitted, that they were always confirmed – which in the eyes of their admirers constituted the strongest argument in favour of these theories. It began to dawn on me that this apparent strength was in fact their weakness.[25]

The mildness of his tone belies the magnitude of his challenge. Indeed, Popper took psychoanalysis as the canonical example of pseudoscience, the type-specimen against which all other possible intellectual frauds should be measured.

Freud didn't help his own case. In 1934, an American psychologist named Saul Rosenzweig wrote to him to inform him of the results of an experiment that seemed to confirm his theory of repression. Freud replied as follows:

> I cannot put much value on these confirmations because the wealth of reliable observations [from the clinical situation] on which these assertions rest, make them independent of experimental verification.[26]

As experiments go, Rosenzweig's was a weak one: it showed only that children are more likely to remember the titles of jigsaw puzzles they have completed compared to those they have failed to solve. Nevertheless, in appearing to suggest that his theories stood on the basis of clinical interpretation alone, Freud's letter defined the attitude of many of his followers when they were challenged to produce anything so drab as experimental evidence. That would prove unfortunate for the future development of the field.

No less regrettable for its standing as an empirical science was the inference that Freud didn't actually think of it as an empirical science at all.

When I trained as a neuropsychologist, the mid-20th-century heyday of psychoanalysis was long gone. Freudian theory had lost the considerable influence it once enjoyed in mainstream mental science. Criticisms had accumulated for decades at a scholarly pace, but now the critiques changed in emotional pitch, and became a bombardment. Popper's tone of mild demurral was gone. Suddenly, the world seemed very *angry* with Freud.

The first serious opposition had come from the behaviourist movement, which tried to rule subjective data out of science altogether, and therefore focused solely on externally observable 'stimuli' and 'responses'. Although this approach began in the 1920s as a methodological strategy, it had morphed by mid-century into a denial that subjective states exist at all. Thus, B. F. Skinner (one of its founders) could declare: 'The "emotions" are excellent examples of the fictional causes to which we commonly attribute behavior'.[27] This was so barmy that it gained traction only in departments of experimental psychology and parts of philosophy. Nobody in the wider cultural world (or psychiatry) took it very seriously.

However, Karl Popper carried enormous intellectual weight. For starters, his Viennese parents were close friends of the Freud family, and Popper himself did voluntary service in a psychoanalytic clinic when he was a university student. In 1919, he joined the Social Democratic Workers' Party of Austria, but subsequently rejected Marxism and all other forms of totalitarianism, and became a vocal supporter of Western liberal democracy. In 1934, he published *The Logic of Scientific Discovery*, in which he first articulated the view that falsifiability is what distinguishes science from non-science. This was his ticket out of Austria, on the eve of the *Anschluss* by Nazi Germany.

After the war, Popper's rise was steep. By 1949, he was professor of logic and scientific method at the London School of Economics, where he lectured and influenced both Imre Lakatos and Paul

Feyerabend, two of the next generation's foremost philosophers of science. By 1959 he was president of the Aristotelian Society, one of the oldest and most prestigious philosophical organizations in the world: a suitable berth for the self-appointed arbiter of science. He readied his strike on Freud – and its echoes resounded down the years.

In the wake of Popper's 1963 attack, the psychometrician Paul Kline published *Fact and Fantasy in Freudian Theory* (1972), an encyclopaedic survey of the research to date. It showed that some parts could be and had been falsified, according to Popper's criterion, but others hadn't been, even after the relevant tests, and therefore remained provisionally true. The body of research that Kline reviewed utilized many non-clinical, experimental methods of the kind that Freud supposedly did not think relevant, and Kline concluded that the jury was still out.

In similarly serious vein, the philologist Sebastiano Timpanaro published *The Freudian Slip: Psychoanalysis and Textual Criticism* (1974), arguing that Freud's accounts of unconsciously motivated slips of the tongue (and pen) could be explained equally well or better by means of purely linguistic criteria. Unlike Kline's book, Timpanaro's conclusion was wholly negative, but it was based on reasonable evidence. Likewise *Freud: Biologist of the Mind* (1979), an intellectual biography by the psychologist and historian of science Frank Sulloway, titled after a description that Freud gave himself. Sulloway claimed that many of Freud's core theories incorporated, or were even derived from, now-discredited 19th-century biological assumptions. Again, this was fair comment. For example, Freud took literally Haeckel's biogenetic law, which claimed that 'ontogeny recapitulates phylogeny' (i.e., that the foetus recapitulates in its anatomical development the whole of evolutionary history, from amoeba to primates via fish and reptile-like forms). Likewise, he was an enthusiastic supporter of Lamarckian theory – according to which we inherit what was learnt by our ancestors. In those respects, he was indeed a creature of his times.

But then the tone darkened. In 1982, a *Rolling Stone* magazine correspondent named Peter Swales published an article, the title of which purported to cast 'New Light on the Origins of Psychoanalysis', by claiming that Freud had had a secret affair with his wife's younger sister and arranged for her to have an abortion. Swales drew attention also to Freud's use of cocaine. (As an early-career scientist, Freud alerted European doctors to the potential medicinal properties of cocaine; he correctly predicted that it might be a potent local anaesthetic and suggested that it might be deployed as an antidepressant, but his recommendation of its use to assist opiate withdrawal proved very unwise.)

Swales's article did not appear in an academic journal, but it laid the foundations for a more serious study, written by the medical historian Elizabeth Thornton. *The Freudian Fallacy: Freud and Cocaine* (1983) argued that Freud's theories resulted from drug-induced derangement: 'Freud was addicted to cocaine throughout the period when his central theories of the unconscious mind and child sexuality were formulated.'

One year earlier, a journalist named Karin Obholzer had published *The Wolf Man: Sixty Years Later* (1982), which showed that the outcome of Freud's treatment of one of his most famous patients was anything but impressive. To Obholzer's delight, and at her instigation, despite the fact that this patient had been generously looked after all his life by members of the psychoanalytic establishment (about which I will have more to say later), the elderly Wolf Man, who always enjoyed the limelight, happily denounced his late analyst.

This paved the way for a book by Jeffrey Masson: *Freud: The Assault on Truth* (1984). Given his position as director of the Sigmund Freud Archives at the US Library of Congress, Masson wrote with special authority. He claimed that Freud had deliberately concealed the fact that childhood sexual abuse was the cause of adult mental illness, insisting instead that his patients' memories of such abuse were fantasies about events which never happened. Strangely, a well-known experimental psychologist named Elizabeth Loftus then used the opposite argument to further undermine Freud's reputation. In *The Myth of Repressed Memory: False Memories and Allegations of Sexual Abuse* (1994), she 'reveal[ed] that despite decades of research, there is absolutely no controlled scientific support for the idea that memories of trauma are routinely banished into the unconscious and then reliably recovered years later'. This seems rather unfair on Freud, who openly published his initial finding that sexual trauma was the typical cause of psychopathology, and then equally openly corrected himself when he realized that this wasn't true for all cases. In other words, Loftus triumphantly 'revealed' what Freud himself had said a century earlier, namely that the memories of sexual abuse reported by (some of) his patients turned out to be false.

Immediately following Masson's book, another distinguished experimental psychologist, Hans Eysenck, published *Decline and Fall of the Freudian Empire* (1985). This argued – as if Kline's (1972) survey of the evidence had never happened – that Freud's speculative theories were only now being subjected to rigorous empirical challenge, and in all areas where such testing had been carried out, they had been falsified completely. (Eysenck himself later fell into scandal. As of 2025, there have been at least 14 retractions of his scientific journal articles and 71 formal expressions of concern about the veracity of his published research findings.)

In 1998, Frederick Crews edited *Unauthorized Freud: Doubters Confront a Legend*, which 'musters 18 opposition stalwarts who accuse the master of being a dogmatist who browbeat his patients and consistently failed to distinguish between their fantasies and his own'. In 1995, Richard Webster published *Why Freud Was Wrong: Sin, Science and Psychoanalysis*, whose title gives a fair indication of its content. Ditto Louis Breger's (2000) *Freud: Darkness in the Midst of Vision*. In 2017, the publishers of Crews' next missive, *Freud: The Making of an Illusion*, claimed that this book 'will stand as the last word on one of the most significant and contested figures of the twentieth century'.* On its cover, it looked as though a capital 'A' had been scribbled over Freud's

---

* Three years later the same house, Profile Books, published my own book, *The Hidden Spring*, which had several favourable words to say about Freud.

name, correcting it to 'FRAUD', though it equally could have been intended as a devil horn.

I have focused here upon what was said about Freud in books from the early 1970s onwards. The same fall-narrative replicates in other popular media: magazines, newspapers, television and radio, and indeed, as we will see, in the scientific literature. I'm not sure why. Newton and Darwin, to pick figures of comparable prominence, got some things wrong and failed to understand others. No one thinks that Newtonian physics is literally true as a final account of reality. Darwin had no idea how inheritance worked in practice. They did the best they could with the tools available to them, and their work has since been modified almost beyond recognition. None of that has damaged their standing as scientific pioneers; whatever controversies may still attach to them, scholars don't generally try to write them out of intellectual history. By contrast, take a look at Allen Esterson's *Seductive Mirage: An Exploration of the Work of Sigmund Freud* (1993); an indictment that 'builds irresistibly to a "proof beyond reasonable doubt" that Freud's claim to rank as a major thinker is unfounded, and indeed quite preposterous'.

Critics of psychoanalysis often find it irritating when, in place of rebuttals, their claims are greeted with diagnoses, as if their viewing the whole thing as a scam just proves how emotionally maladjusted they are. You will have to take it on trust that such a deflection is not my intent when I observe that many of the authors just cited were at one time admirers of Freud, and that many of their attacks seem to suggest a zeal, almost a fury, to expose the imposter. It is not under the flag of any particular theory that I pose the question whether such stances might indicate a deeper, more interesting feeling of betrayal than the case warrants – even if, for the sake of argument, we were to grant all the faults they allege.

At any rate, my Freud is not theirs. He differs also in important respects from the quasi-spiritual master who presides over the scattered schools of psychoanalysis that have survived the waning of his star. I was a neuropsychologist first and a Freudian analyst second. For several decades I have practised clinically in both capacities, as well as at the interface between them. I have published a good deal of scientific research in both fields. Recently, I discharged my duties as the official translator of Freud's complete psychological works. That took 29 years of toil, during which I immersed myself in the progression of his thought quite thoroughly.

I mention all this not to claim any final authority, but only to ask a serious hearing. In my estimation, Freud was a scientist, and a very good one. Just as Luria was secretly doing psychoanalysis the whole time that he was laying the foundations of neuropsychology, I believe that Freud was doing what amounted to quasi-neuropsychology from the beginning of his career to its end. He pursued his inquiries in the informal way that he did because no other was open to him. Nevertheless, his theories were always intended to be answerable to the full range of empirical evidence, and ultimately to rejoin the rest of medical science. Now is the time to see how they fare.

In the past century, neuropsychology has amassed vast amounts of data. New imaging tools have pushed the frontiers of observability far beneath the surface of the living brain, and many of Freud's conjectures have withered under their glare. Yet his deepest, broadest ideas have held up remarkably well. The field that Luria built is no longer such a young science – yet after 50 more years of intensive work since his death, its best model of the mind looks very like one that he would have recognized from his first reading of Freud – perhaps especially when it comes to the three chapters that he declined to write.

None of this means that Freud was *right*, of course. As Popper correctly taught, the most obvious pattern might not be the real one. But it suggests that psychoanalysis, as Freud conceived of it, should be taken seriously. It suggests that, however limited his methods, they might indeed have guided him to a part of the truth, and quite a large one at that. Most strikingly, when we look at the puzzles that still haunt neuroscience and psychological medicine – psychiatry in particular – from a Freudian perspective, important things seem to fall into place. And if Freud *was* right, it is clear that a lot of things we are doing at present are wrong, and will have to change.

Speaking now as a psychoanalyst, that is always an interesting place to be.

CHAPTER TWO
The Interpretation of Dreams

ANALYST: What is the craving like?
PATIENT: It's just not regulated. I lie down to watch TV. Then I need to eat. Then I'll pick at this, pick at that – kind of like a buffet. Then I think: 'You have to be careful.' It's a real challenge. But there's also a feeling of freedom to enjoy something. I love the freedom. It's something about the tasting. I can't name it. It's the whole experience. I imagine it's like when people cut themselves. There's a feedback loop. There's a ravenous aspect, but it's not that I'm hungry. It seems to stand in for something else. It's also something about the need to be adventurous. To go find the food; to go out and find something new and bring it back. I always want to try something new.
ANALYST: You said that you feel the same kind of excitement sexually?
PATIENT: Yeah. I think there is a crossover. But I'm not sure in which direction. There is the same voraciousness.

— *From the author's clinical files*

When I first started studying the brain, I became interested in a rare genetic condition called Urbach–Wiethe disease, named after the two Viennese doctors who first described it in 1929. It causes skin abnormalities and hoarseness of voice, but also calcium deposits in an almond-shaped part of the brain located just beneath the ears – the 'amygdala' (meaning almond) – which is largely responsible for the emotion of fear. Only 400 or so cases have been reported in the medical literature. A substantial proportion of those, however, come from a small town called Springbok, near where I was born.

In Springbok, in a very isolated community in which inbreeding is common, it affects about one in 12 individuals. Once these patients reach puberty, they show a striking reduction in anxiety. In fact, they are utterly fearless, to a dangerous degree. The most celebrated case is the American patient known as SM. Over the course of her life, she was the victim of numerous traumatic crimes and life-threatening encounters. She got held up both at knifepoint and gunpoint, and was almost killed in a domestic violence incident, but she did not exhibit any signs of desperation and urgency, or any of the other behavioural responses that would normally confirm the traumatic nature of these events. In an experiment[1] she displayed no fear at all in response to handling snakes and spiders, walking through a fairground haunted house, or watching fear-inducing film clips, although she felt all the other expected emotions, such as interest, curiosity and excitement. 'Because SM is missing her amygdala, she doesn't have this cascade of responses that comprise a state of fear,' the neurologist who examined her said. 'And because of that, she's unable to feel fear.'[2]

One of my own patients with this condition, Paulina Z, was a young woman roughly my own age. Born in Springbok, she had a harrowing history of childhood abuse at the hands of her alcoholic father – not an uncommon story in this very poor and marginalized community. During an investigation that I conducted as part of a research project, she told me that an *advantage* of her disease was that – since the onset of her symptoms at puberty – she no longer experienced the nightmares that used to plague her. How does it happen, I thought, that damage to less than one cubic centimetre of tissue on either side of the brain can relieve someone from a lifetime of bad dreams? I asked the other participants in my project about their dreams, too. They all reported the same thing: no nightmares since the onset of their skin and voice problems.

Instead, the dreams they reported were short, simple and wishful, like children's dreams. One patient said that she saw her deceased father, which made her happy. Another said that she dreamt her disabled daughter could walk. Another reported that he was lying under a beautiful bush, laden with the most delicious fruit he had ever eaten. Another – who was unemployed – dreamt that he found a job. Another, that she was on a bus, going on a holiday, something she had done only once before in her life.

At the time, I had no particular interest in psychoanalysis, and didn't know about Freud's wish-fulfilment theory. Still, what these patients said very much intrigued me. I began raising the subject with patients with different neurological conditions. It seemed reasonable to expect that, just like the Urbach–Wiethe sufferers, people who had lost a certain mental capacity in their waking life would report the same impairment in their dreams.

In some cases, that is indeed what I found. A man who had lost colour vision due to carbon monoxide poisoning dreamed in black and white. A man who had lost the ability to recognize familiar faces following a brain tumour couldn't recognize faces in his dreams, though he knew his late mother in a dream by her voice.

Other disorders seemed to work differently, though. A patient who was blinded by a stroke in his visual cortex reported to me that he could still see in his dreams. The same applied to patients who had lost the power of speech due to damage in Broca's area: all of them reported that they could still speak fluently in their dreams. These patients' right arms are typically paralysed, so I asked them about that, too, and all six of them told me they could still move the arm in their dreams. The same applied to patients with paraplegia caused by injuries to the spinal cord: they could walk normally in their dreams. More than one of them spoke to me of their repeated disappointment, upon waking, to find that it was 'just a dream'.

These disparities struck me as so odd that I embarked upon a systematic study of how damage to different brain structures affects dreaming. In outline, this was the same type of research that the pioneers of neuropsychology had undertaken with respect to language, memory, perception, attention, skilled movement and so on. You examine the patient clinically to discover how their psychological capabilities and experiences have altered, then you identify which parts of their brains are diseased or damaged, and you start to assign component mental functions to the different parts on the basis of these correlations. (Thankfully, in the era of brain imaging, one no longer needs to wait for the patient's death and autopsy.) For example, as Luria taught us, once you have identified the different ways in which language is impaired by damage to the different parts of the brain, you have identified the multiple components of the 'functional system' for language.

Because dreams are so difficult to study scientifically (since they are retrospective, subjective descriptions of notoriously confusing and forgettable hallucinatory episodes that occur during sleep), it turned out that no one had got around to looking at them in this standard fashion. My way around the problem of subjective reports was to study a sufficiently large number of patients (361 in total), which meant that I could collect dream reports from *groups* of them with damage to the same brain regions. There is no denying that dreams are fleeting and fugitive phenomena, but even allowing for that, if all the people in an anatomical group report the same change in their dreams, why not believe them? This study (which I began in 1985) became my doctoral thesis. Insofar as it has been investigated psychologically, the phenomenon of beginner's luck is now regarded as being largely an illusion. That is a consoling thought for me, because I have never, in my long and often satisfying career, stumbled on anything quite as big as the discoveries that emerged in the course of that research.

The leading theory of dreams at that time was developed by Allan Hobson, a professor of neurophysiology at Harvard. Using electroencephalography (EEG) combined with sleep awakening, it had been discovered in the 1950s that dreaming – a psychological state – almost always occurs during the rapid-eye-movement (REM) phase of the sleep cycle, a physiological state.[3] This correlation led neuroscientists in the 1960s to search for the part of the brain that generates REM sleep, since that part presumably also generated dreams, given how tightly correlated the two states were.

After a difficult search, they found the REM generator in the brainstem (literally, the stalk at the bottom of the brain that connects it to the spinal cord).[4] Hobson's research showed that one small part of the brainstem, the 'mesopontine tegmentum', emitted a special chemical in a roughly 90-minute cycle during sleep, and that this triggered the REM phase. He therefore inferred that dreaming itself was caused by this chemical, a neuromodulator called acetylcholine, activating the cortex of the brain.

In his book *The Dreaming Brain* (1988), Hobson claimed that these experimental findings disproved Freudian theory. After all, if dreams were caused by the lowly brainstem releasing 'motivationally neutral'[5] chemicals – on a timer, no less – there could be little left for the noble cortex of the forebrain to do. Yet that was where ideas lived. Therefore, Hobson wrote:

> If we assume that the physiological substrate of consciousness is in the forebrain, these facts completely eliminate any possible contribution of ideas (or their neural substrate) to the primary driving force of the dream process.[6]

Freud's theory that dreams were the products of wishes turned out to be falsifiable after all. Indeed, it turned out to be false; for what are wishes if not ideas? Hobson concluded that dreaming served no purpose: it was 'an epiphenomenon of REM sleep', standing in much the same relation to the real dynamics of the sleeping brain as your shadow does to the movements of your body.[7]

The correlation between REM sleep and dreaming was established by non-invasive methods. In this case, by the sleep EEG method: patients went to bed wearing a sort of electrical shower cap that measured their brain's activation levels. That might sound invasive in the sense that few would choose to sleep that way, but everything is relative: compared to how the link was established between REM sleep and the mesopontine tegmentum, it wasn't so bad.

The latter research required systematic and deliberate damage to the brains of hundreds of experimental subjects. How else could one determine which lesions, in particular, prevented the subject from entering REM sleep? For this reason, the research was conducted, not on humans, but on cats and rats. Cats and rats can't report their experiences at the best of times, and certainly not when their brains are riddled with surgical incisions. In this experimental format, then, there could be no question of monitoring the presence of dreaming itself. The subjective side of the equation had to be, as it were, taken on faith.

Unlike Michel Jouvet, the neuroscientist who conducted most of the research just mentioned, I did my doctoral research on human subjects who had sustained naturally-occurring brain lesions.[8] I had access to large numbers of them because there were only three neuropsychologists in the whole of Johannesburg, a city of 2 million people at that time (now closer to 6 million). I decided to study human beings rather than cats and rats for the obvious reason that I wanted to correlate damage in the different parts of the brain with changes in *dreaming* – a subjective state, which requires verbal reports – not changes in REM sleep – an objective state, which does not. The fact that my research subjects could report their experienced dream states led me to two surprising discoveries.

Firstly, patients with damage to the mesopontine tegmentum, who no longer display REM sleep, continue to experience dreams, while patients with damage elsewhere in the brain, who no longer experience dreams, continue to display REM sleep. This is called a 'double dissociation of function': it demonstrates that the mechanism which produces REM sleep cannot be the same as the one which produces dreaming, since abolition of the first mechanism has no effect upon the second one, and vice-versa.

The other thing I found was the brain structure that *does* generate dreams.

The culprit turned out to be a massive fibre pathway arising from the brainstem and running upward toward the eyes, through the lower half of the forebrain. It is called the medial forebrain bundle, and it contains the 'mesocortical-mesolimbic' dopamine circuit. Hobson made much of the fact that acetylcholine is 'motivationally neutral' in his repudiation of the wishfulness of dreams. The same cannot be said of dopamine. Ever since it was discovered in the 1950s, this dopamine circuit has been known as 'the brain's reward system'.[9] The pioneering neuroscientist of emotion, Jaak Panksepp, named it the SEEKING system. His colleague Kent Berridge called it the 'wanting' system.

When Popper asserted that, to qualify as scientific, a theory must in principle be falsifiable, he took Freud's claim about the wishfulness of dreams as his paradigmatic example of a theory that didn't meet that standard. Allan Hobson was certainly no enthusiast of Freud's,* yet he paid him the compliment of insisting that his theory not only *could* be falsified by experiment, but that he, Hobson, had falsified it. He had shown how dreaming really worked, and how wishing had nothing to do with it.

This left me in an odd position. After reading Hobson's arguments, I was persuaded that Freud's theory *could have been* falsified (albeit using different methods than Freud used); yet, on the basis of my own fortuitous discoveries, I knew that the actual evidence failed to refute him. Instead, it seemed to me that it was Hobson's rival explanation that had fallen to the test of falsification. Not only that, but the real origin of dreaming in the brain seemed to provide, well . . . 'confirmation' is a banned word in Popperian philosophy of science, so let's say that, if the brain's dopamine reward system really did generate dreaming, that looked good for the wish-fulfilment theory. Indeed, it was starting to look like Freud's theory might contain some residue of science after all.

---

* Here is a representative quote: 'Not only was Freud's dream theory wrong, but psychoanalysis has systematically warped psychology and delayed the development of psychiatry' (Hobson, 2011).

At that time, it was hard to find any medical scientists who still taught Freud. The psychiatrists at the medical school of my own university – the University of the Witwatersrand, Johannesburg – were ruthlessly reductionistic. They treated emotional disorders pharmacologically, and they enthusiastically deployed electro-convulsive therapy with depressed patients who did not respond to such drugs, a horrible treatment to witness. As a last resort, therefore, I attended a series of open seminars (open to postgraduate students from any faculty) led by a professor of Comparative Literature.

His name was Jean-Pierre de la Porte, and he was interested in the history of ideas. At first I found it hard to take him seriously. He was an Afrikaner who feigned a thick French accent, and had changed his name accordingly. A strange fish. All the same, it was from him that I learnt that Freud had been a pioneering neuroscientist who contributed to the discovery of the neuron and to the mapping of the internal connectivity of the human brainstem. This Freud had also been a clinical neurologist who made fundamental contributions to our understanding of the cerebral palsies, and a neuropsychologist-before-the-letter who published a breakthrough book on the brain mechanisms of language. In fact, it was only when Freud was in his forties and his medical career was well underway that he started to sound recognizably like a psychoanalyst.

It happened in a momentous paper with an unassuming title: 'Some Points of Comparison between Organic and Hysterical Motor Paralyses' (1893). Freud was trying to work out why disturbing ideas sometimes produce bodily symptoms. Using the example of hysterical paralysis of the arm, he pointed out that the distribution of such a paralysis in the body corresponded not to the way the arm is controlled by and represented anatomically in the cortex of the brain, but rather to the *idea* of an arm. In hysterical paralysis (in this example), the upper limb is typically affected equally from hand to shoulder, whereas in paralysis due to brain damage, the hand is typically more paralysed than the elbow, which in turn is more paralysed than the shoulder, and there is some paralysis of the facial muscles too. This is because a much larger region of the motor cortex represents the hand than does the elbow and the shoulder, and the region for the hand merges into the region for the face. If the whole arm is equally paralysed, and the face is completely unaffected, the cause is highly unlikely to be damage to its cortical control centre. It must be some association with the *idea* of the arm – i.e., with the thing represented by the word 'arm' – depicted in the imagination from shoulder to hand.

On this basis, Freud concluded that what at first sight appeared to be the product of damage to the tissues of the brain must instead result from what he called 'the lesion of an idea' – a pathological association between thoughts. Given what I knew about the anatomy of the motor cortex, and my clinical experience with cortical paralysis, that struck me as a good argument.

Later in the same article, Freud argued that the pathogenic ideas in question were associated with strong *emotions*. Specifically, he argued that hysterical disorders (we now call them 'functional neurological disorders') arose from the connection between thoughts and feelings; that they arose from the ideas that patients used to *regulate* their feelings. Thus, for example, hysterical paralysis of the arm might follow from a suppressed memory of something that the patient previously did with that arm. Freud used the analogy of someone who has shaken hands with the Emperor, not wanting to break that association by washing the hand. (He was not yet a psychoanalyst, so he didn't use the more suggestive example of something embarrassingly sexual that a patient might have done with their hand.)

Based on what I knew at the time, I found all of this surprisingly persuasive. It made a kind of overall logical sense; and in an odd way it spoke to my own feelings, promising relief, if not from paralysis, then certainly from a kind of numb detachment.

As it happens, the mystery of how a brain injury could turn one person into another person was why I was interested in the brain in the first place. When I was a child, my elder brother Lee fell off a building, sustaining a serious head injury. It changed him permanently. He lost his developmental milestones; it was as if my admired big brother had become my embarrassing little brother. I was haunted by the questions this left me with. What *is* a mind? How does it arise within the body, and make people who they are? Indeed, what makes us free agents instead of inanimate matter, or mere automata? What I had learned as a student neuropsychologist was so remote from anything that I might recognize as an answer to those questions that the questions themselves seemed to go into a state of suspended animation. I was studying neuropsychology in the orthodox way, not wanting to do anything that would frighten the horses, but it wasn't getting me any closer to the burning mysteries that drew me to the field in the first place.

When I discovered Freud, I remembered why I wanted to be a neuropsychologist. On the strength of what I learned in those seminars with de la Porte, and the further readings that he spurred, I made an unusual decision: to supplement my just-completed training in neuropsychology with a further qualification, as a psychoanalyst.

The professor of neurosurgery in Johannesburg at that time was Robert Lipschitz. He was a fellow of the Royal College of Surgeons of Edinburgh, and he drove a vintage Rolls Royce Silver Shadow that took up two spaces in our crowded hospital parking garage. When I told him that I was moving to London to train in psychoanalysis, he was dismayed. 'Don't you know that they start out as patients and then work their way up?'

Despite his misgivings, Lipschitz sent word to a neurosurgeon whom he had trained in Johannesburg, now a consultant in London, asking him to help me when I got there. This man duly introduced me to the professor of neurosurgery at the Royal London Hospital in Whitechapel.* After a 15-minute chat, and

---

*John Hughlings Jackson, who influenced both Freud and Luria greatly, had worked there in the 1860s.

an inaugural lecture on 'The Shortcomings of the Psychometric Approach to Neuropsychology', I had a job.

This sounds like an old boys' network, and no doubt that's largely what it was. Viewed from the perspective of a white South African, there was a good deal about the set-up at the Royal London Hospital in those days that felt unsettlingly familiar. The professors and consultants – who always sat, wearing dark suits, in the front rows of the historic lecture theatres in which working-class patients were displayed for teaching purposes – spoke Oxbridge English. The residents and housemen (as they were called) spoke with the full range of regional British accents, and they always sat at the back, in a motley mish-mash of clothing. How does it happen, I wondered, that the ones with those accents and clothes never get to be consultants and professors? Still, for whatever reason – whether it was because people with colonial accents were exempted from this silly English game, or because my sponsor had explained that I came from a 'good' family back home – I was happy to be included in the front rows.

Like many jokes, Lipschitz's quip about psychoanalysts was simply true. The first requirement of a trainee psychoanalyst is still that they must undergo analysis themselves. After a minimum of one year's treatment, they may begin attending theoretical seminars. And so, for several years, I lived a Jekyll-and-Hyde existence. Every morning, before going to the hospital where I practised neuropsychology in the neurosurgery and neurology wards, and pursued my neuroscientific research interests, I spent a 50-minute hour lying on the couch of a psychoanalyst at the Anna Freud Centre in Hampstead; a long way (in every sense of the word) from Whitechapel.

My analyst was a Yorkshireman named Clifford Yorke. He had been wounded while serving in the British medical corps during the war and now he walked with a limp. After the war, he served as psychiatrist-in-charge at the Hampstead Clinic, as the Anna Freud Centre was then called, succeeding Anna Freud as its director when she retired in 1978. Anna was Sigmund's daughter.

The psychoanalytic lineage from Freud to me could not have been more direct.

Clifford Yorke explained the fundamentals: I must lie on his couch, five times per week for 50 minutes at a time, and say everything that came into my head; everything, without exception, including things that seemed irrelevant and nonsensical, and especially things that would normally be considered inappropriate to talk about, such as my feeling that it was creepy to be analysed by this old soldier with a limp, that I didn't want to think about what his leg looked like under his trousers, that I didn't want to picture him in the privacy of his bathroom, but in fact I was, vividly. This is called the 'fundamental rule' of psychoanalysis: an injunction to report *everything*. It is the essence of the method of 'free association'. Dr Yorke warned me that he would remain silent for the most part, interrupting my monologues only to note significant patterns that might emerge, possibly revealing something about what lay behind my associations. (For that reason, sadly, he never shared his personal memories of Anna Freud with me.)

Over the next few weeks and months of disciplined rambling, patterns did indeed come into view. I dreamt that I was looking for a letter that my late father had left for me – written just before he underwent the heart surgery that killed him – a letter that could tell me where he had hidden his love for me. I wanted to find that letter. When I reported this dream to Dr Yorke, I was suddenly overcome by sadness and regret, and I started to sob. My mixed feelings about Clifford Yorke resembled those that I had had about my father, the taciturn and undemonstrative boss of a diamond mine. And yet it was only now that Yorke had pointed out this 'transference' from my father onto him that I became fully aware of the childhood feelings. I knew that there was something of substance in my father, something that he could have shared with me, perhaps some important insight about life that I could have learnt from him, and been grateful for and felt proud of – something I wanted to identify with and believe in. But I despaired of ever receiving it.

A few months into my analysis, my wife asked me: 'Why are you limping?' She was right; I was dragging my right leg, just like Clifford Yorke: a concrete enactment of my identification with him, and of my wish to be with him, standing in for my unreachable father.

The most peculiar thing that happened during my analysis, however, was my recovery of a very early memory. One day, while talking about the experience of my brother's return from hospital, I had an uncanny recollection of being in hospital myself. I was inside a translucent bubble of some kind, and I felt lost and disorientated: there was a constant low-level glow surrounding the bubble, which made it impossible to tell whether it was day or night.

When I got home from work, I phoned my mother in South Africa and asked her if I had ever been in a hospital, encased in something like a plastic sphere. 'Of course,' she replied. At the age of two I had been admitted to a high-care unit with double pneumonia. I was in the hospital for two weeks, and in an oxygen tent for several days. It had been a difficult time, my mother explained, in part because the hospital barred parents from visiting, as it would 'only upset the child'.

In the psychoanalytic sessions that followed, further details of my hospitalization came back to me. I'd remembered nothing about the entire episode before, so I remarked that I must have 'repressed' it. To this, Dr Yorke replied that it was not repressed, since I could remember it. Repressed memories can *never* be remembered – by definition – he explained; they can only be inferred.

He went on to describe an experience of his own. Some years ago, he was watching a television documentary which included a scene from a Nazi concentration camp. The camera panned across a sign in German. At that moment, he realized: 'I was there.' And true enough, he had been: he was part of the group that liberated the Bergen-Belsen death camp. He had always known this fact but, he explained, he had never recalled the experience. 'It was a scene so horrific, it was beyond imagination. Quite unlike anything else I have experienced before or since.'

He said that such instances (his experience and mine) of forgetting-despite-remembering should probably be understood as 'state-dependent' memory phenomena, rather than as instances of repression. It is well established that people are better able to recall things when they are in the same emotional state as they were when the original experience occurred.

I was touched by his telling me this personal story and his explaining this bit of theory. It is something he almost never did; a rare enactment (in the 'countertransference', as they call it) of my wish that my father might take me into his confidence.

And so, my analysis continued in its own peculiar way, day after day. The fabric of my life was unpicked, knots and all, and then rewoven in a less precarious fashion. I obeyed the fundamental rule as diligently as I could, reporting every thought and feeling that passed by the train-window of my mind. One day, doing so, I realized that I was speaking into a void. Clifford Yorke had fallen asleep. (In fairness to him, he had just undergone hip-replacement surgery.) I was enraged. There I was, trying to convey every detail of what was occurring to me, as instructed – no matter how unedifying – and my supposed analyst wasn't even listening. When the flush of anger subsided, I reflected on what had happened, and found myself again remembering the oxygen tent, and how lost I had felt.

I can't convey some of the most important things that happened in my analysis. Not only because I don't want to (a significant point in itself) but because I *can't*, in the way that you can't recall a dream. There's a special irony in the fact that some of the basic ingredients of the talking cure can't be communicated in words. What I can tell you is that, along the way, one of my most troubling symptoms disappeared. This was severe death anxiety. Ever since my brother's accident, I had been miserably preoccupied by the fact of mortality. Now, the symptom had somehow lost its premise. Of its own accord, my fear went away. I was free to live.

In 1988, almost a decade after it was published, I read Frank Sulloway's critical biography, *Freud: Biologist of the Mind*.[10] (I read a lot of books about Freud in the wake of de la Porte's seminar.) In a footnote, Sulloway claimed that the reason so few people appreciated the importance of Freud's neuroscientific work was that his 'pre-analytical' writings were never translated into English. This would soon change, he said: a four-volume edition was about to be issued under the editorship of Erwin Stengel.

Assuming that this edition must now be available, I ordered it through a local academic bookseller in Johannesburg. When it didn't arrive, my bookseller wrote to the publisher, only to learn that the edition had been cancelled. The editor had died on the job.

That was, of course, frustrating, but I didn't give up hope. When I moved to London the following year, I arranged to meet with the publisher. He showed me two box files containing Stengel's drafts. It had proven impossible to find a replacement editor, he lamented, since any viable candidate must be competent not only in German and psychoanalysis, but also in neuroscience. I was already two of those things: since I was born in the district of Lüderitz in Namibia, a former German colony, I was a German-speaking neuroscientist, and I was about to train in psychoanalysis. We shook hands, and with that I accepted my promotion, from being a prospective buyer of *The Complete Neuroscientific Works of Sigmund Freud*, to being its editor and translator.

It quickly became apparent that Stengel's translations were shoddy, and that he had overlooked a huge number of Freud's neuroscientific papers: more than 200 omissions, published between 1877 and 1900. I collected all the original works together and set about translating them afresh. Sulloway turned out to be right about one thing: *it is difficult to appreciate the scientific foundations of Freud's theories without reading these works*. I will trace just one of the threads, to illustrate this point.

In the late 1870s and early 1880s, Freud was working with cutting-edge neural imaging technology: powerful microscopes. (His own best instrument was a 'Hartnack No. 10', a highly regarded device with a water-immersion lens and a $1/16$ th-inch focal length.) In an 1882 article concerning the structure of nerve cells in the crayfish, published almost a decade before the discovery of the neuron, Freud cast doubt on the prevailing theory that nerve fibres merely 'pass through' nerve cells.[11] The structural relation between nerve fibres and cells, which are now understood to form a single unit called the neuron, was still completely unknown. Yet in a manuscript that he started writing three years later – a textbook on neuroanatomy that he never published* – Freud remarked that 'we must consider the interruption of a nervous pathway [the fibres] by grey matter [the cells] to have consequences for what it conducts'.[12] He decided that it must be the grey junctions that determine the pattern of connectivity in the nervous system, not the white fibres that seemingly pass through them.

Building upon this insight a few years later, Freud turned against the authoritative view of his teacher, the neuroanatomist and psychiatrist Theodor Meynert, to the effect that stimuli are 'projected' directly from the sense organs onto the grey matter of the cortex via the white matter of the nerves. Freud's alternative view was that sensory stimuli are represented indirectly and repeatedly within the brain, rather than simply projected onto its cortex. Here, the idea that he took issue with might seem rather puzzling in its own right. That's partly because, in a digital age, it takes an effort to recover the naivety of an analogue model. Think of how patterns of light pass through the lens of a microscope. You could also think of how soundwaves vibrate a stylus that cuts a groove that vibrates a stylus that produces a soundwave of more or less the same 'shape' as the one it started with; the conducting medium might flip or rotate, expand or shrink the original impression, but the basic pattern ought to survive these merely

---

* Freud seems to have lost his nerve. He wrote the following to his fiancée on December 7, 1885: 'Only one thing speaks against this undertaking, namely that it is audacious, that it must be covered by a great name, and that I therefore dare not allow it to be published under mine. Nevertheless, I will still write it.'

'topological' distortions. Similarly, if nerve fibres conducted impressions more or less unaltered from the eye (or any other sense organ) to the brain, then why suppose that the images formed in our consciousness could be anything other than topologically faithful analogue recordings of the outside world as it presents itself to our senses?

Yet the sensory pathways, Freud observed, were repeatedly interrupted by clumps of grey matter. Surely, he argued, these interruptions must alter the nature of the information that emerges on the other side. And so:

> The first task of brain anatomy is to distinguish the bundles [of fibres] exiting the individual grey substances and to discover their course and destination. The continuation of a bundle, in the physiological sense, can be any other bundle that exits the same grey substance. Any bundle can therefore have a large number of 'continuations' which subsequently conduct the impulses emanating from it.[13]

What Freud was saying here in 1888 was that the actual structure of the nervous system made it unreasonable to assume a direct route from the sense organs to the cortex, and thus to infer the literal projection of images from A to B. Instead, he argued, the images seemed to fracture into multiple bits, and these derivatives *represent and re-represent* the originals in widely dispersed brain regions rather than *project* them onto the cortex.

Three years later, in his (1891) book about the brain mechanisms of language, Freud made the same point. Now, however, he shifted from anatomical to functional terms: 'We cannot but assume that the *functional* significance of a fibre en route to the cerebral cortex has changed each time it emerges anew from a grey mass'.[14] He continued, in a passage so inspired that I sometimes find myself looking it up again, just to confirm that it is real:

> We know only that the fibres which reach the cerebral cortex after their progression through other grey tissues still maintain

some relationship to the periphery of the body, but they can no longer deliver an image which resembles it topologically [i.e., which literally 'projects' it]. They contain the body periphery in the same way as – to borrow an example from the subject with which we are concerned here [i.e., language] – a poem contains the alphabet, in a complete rearrangement, serving different purposes, with manifold links between the individual topological elements, whereby some of them may be rendered several times, others not at all. If it were possible to trace in detail this rearrangement which takes place from the level of the spinal projection up to the cerebral cortex, one would probably find that the governing principle is purely functional, and that topographic relations are maintained only in so far as they fit in with the claims of function. As there is no indication that this rearrangement is reversed in the cerebral cortex to produce a topographically complete projection, we may suppose that, in general, the body periphery is *no longer contained topologically* in the higher parts of the brain, including the cortex, *but only functionally*.[15]

I think it is fair to say that this represents the very moment when psychoanalysis was born. By looking at the branching of the neural pathways that link the sense organs to the brain, Freud inferred that our impressions of the world must be chopped up and rearranged in all manner of ways before they form our conscious experience. What happens during that labyrinthine journey between periphery and centre, between the nerve terminals in a limb and the idea of the limb, between body and mind? What poems might our brains be composing from the alphabet of raw sensations, and according to which mysterious rules of transformation?

At the time Freud wrote this passage, not a single technology for studying the dynamics of the living brain existed. (The EEG was introduced toward the end of his life, but its application was interrupted by the Second World War.) Freud never doubted that the brain was the place where our sensory flux becomes conscious experience. In all his surviving papers, published and unpublished, and all the reports his contemporaries made about his stated opinions, there is never any hint of metaphysical dualism – of disembodied mind stuff. He was a scientist, ever the biologist of the mind. Yet the puzzles that his study of hysterical paralysis led him to investigate seemed to imply a level of organization in our mental apparatus that no physiological method was adequate to explore. It was clear that problems could arise without any damage to the tissues of the brain whatsoever. What metaphor could be used to visualize them? (We might think of a virus in a computer. Freud barely knew of traffic in a city.)

After he rejected Meynert's naive speculations about sensory images being deposited in cortical cells, Freud shifted allegiance to a rival current in neurology. The French school, led by Jean-Martin Charcot, prioritized clinical observation over physiological speculation, but even Charcot saw his approach as an interim strategy only. It was just a matter of time, he asserted, before technical advances in neuropathology would make it possible for us to visualize 'dynamic lesions' in the brain which produced hysterical paralyses and the like.

Freud had a different idea – and, I have to say, a better one.

In the breakthrough (1893) paper in which he first claimed that these seemingly physical disabilities must be caused by 'lesions of ideas', he put the point in dogmatic terms. Charcot's prediction that it would someday be possible to visualize 'dynamic lesions' responsible for such disorders, Freud argued, still implied that these lesions were somehow localizable. Behind the notion of dynamic lesions, therefore, he wrote, 'there is hidden the idea of a [physiological] lesion like oedema or anaemia':

> I, on the contrary, assert that the lesion in hysterical paralyses must be completely independent of the anatomy of the nervous system, since *in its paralyses and other manifestations hysteria behaves as though anatomy did not exist or as though it had no knowledge of it*.[16]

One way or another, the physiological route was closed. How, then, should a biologist proceed? When he was studying the nerve cells of crayfish and the spinal cords of lampreys, Freud had rolled up his sleeves and counted nerve fibres. Faced with this new challenge, there was only one thing for it: to start at the other end of the microscope. He would, like Charcot, prioritize clinical observation. Yet rather than waiting for advances in physiology, he would switch to psychology right away. He could study the lesioned *ideas* of his patients directly, and infer from these end-products of the functional labyrinth the rules of transformation that lay behind them. On that basis, he would develop theories about the underlying machinery.

Freud wanted to know what the apparatus of the mind was hiding as it presented itself consciously. What did it do when nobody was looking? How might its workings expose themselves in moments of malfunction? To this end, he explored in depth not only the symptoms and signs of hysteria and other mental disorders (phobias, obsessions, and so on), but also what might be called 'normal' malfunctions: slips of the tongue, momentary forgetting of names, and the errors of logic that make jokes funny. It wasn't enough just to collect, describe and classify specimens of such phenomena. Freud's approach was much the same as Luria's would be to the analysis of neuropsychological syndromes. His aim was to identify the *underlying factors* that explained the full complexity of appearances. These hidden but inferred causes, Freud believed – no matter how long it took him to identify and adequately describe them – would eventually reveal the elementary components of the systems that produce psychopathological syndromes. This, in turn, would reveal nothing less than the laws that govern mental life in its subjective aspect.

Here was a new horizon for science. Various names were tried out for it. Metapsychology (because it probed what lay 'beyond' consciousness). Depth psychology (because it dug up what was 'underneath' it). Psychoanalysis – on the model of chemical analysis – a separating out, a loosening (*lysis*) up (*ana*) of the elemental components of the mind.

And where best to witness our thought processes falling apart?

> There is one psychical product to be met with in the most normal persons, which yet presents a very striking analogy to the wildest productions of insanity, and was no more intelligible to philosophers than insanity itself. I refer to dreams. Psychoanalysis is founded upon the analysis of dreams; the interpretation of dreams is the most complete piece of work the young science has done up to the present.[17]

That, in outline, was the method in Freud's madness. On these foundations he built an edifice of theory that captivated the world and dominated the mental sciences, without serious challenge, for half a century. On these foundations, over the past 130 years, hundreds of thousands of people lay on tens of thousands of couches, producing billions of free associations, granting unfettered access to their innermost thoughts and feelings, in pursuit of the truth about themselves, in the belief that it might relieve them from suffering. From this vast exercise, it was hoped, the yield for humanity would be scientific understanding of the part of nature that Freud called 'psychical reality'. A wish granted as easily and as improbably as the innocent dreams of Paulina Z.

One of the second-generation psychoanalysts that I met in their dotage (a refugee from Hitler's greater Germany) told me a wonderful Weimar joke: *Sogar die Zukunft war früher besser* – 'In the old days, even the future was better.' Who could have predicted what would become of Freud's psychoanalysis?

Throughout human history, the mind (or soul) was the preserve of priests, clerics, moralists, philosophers, healers and the like, people who – despite their diverse perspectives – always pronounced upon how we *should* and *should not* be, feel and think, who exhorted us to some elevated status, above the animals and the rest of nature. So, when Freud proclaimed the human mind to be just another part of nature and subjected it to the same cold, scientific scrutiny that is applied to birds, trees, volcanos, comets and the liver, he committed an outrage: a slap in the face of the pious.

Freud claimed that those who judge do not want to understand. Could it be that the multiple absurd accusations and fantasies about him that proliferated through the 20th century were evoked by his attempt to replace moral judgement with scientific understanding? If he did not actively condemn the animalistic, unethical, blasphemous and immoral side of our nature, then he *was* all those things.

Despite its best efforts, few pursuits are more human than science. Forever falling short of certain knowledge, its products are never more certifiably scientific than when they are overturned. For a long time now, we scientists with the serious stamp have been sure that Freud's efforts were in vain, or worse, vainglorious:

> Whether a man sacrificed his life to rescue a drowning child (a case of sublimation) or whether he murdered the child by drowning (a case of repression) could not possibly be predicted or excluded by Freud's theory.[18]

Then again, as one of his less acknowledged intellectual fathers observed, the timber of humanity is not well suited to the construction of straight things – least of all, paths to truth.[19] As we will discover, the journey in this case was a particularly winding one. So let's jump ahead.

CHAPTER THREE
The Mental Apparatus

> PATIENT: My parents don't give a damn about me. They show no interest in anything I do. None.
> ANALYST: But they did come to your school play last night.
> PATIENT: That was only because they couldn't give a damn not to come.
>
> — *From the author's clinical files*

It is truly striking how committed some observers are to denying that Freud did neuroscience. 'In reality', wrote Matthew Cobb in his panoramic history of neuroscience *The Idea of the Brain* (2020): 'Freud had nothing novel or insightful to say about how the brain works.'

For the most part Cobb's book is rather good, but this is plainly unfair. Even before his turn to psychoanalysis, Freud said many influential things about how the brain works, and some downright prescient ones. A whole chapter in Shepherd's *Foundations of the Neuron Doctrine* (1991) is devoted to his contributions to the discovery of this basic unit of nervous tissue. (The final step was taken by Santiago Ramón y Cajal, who used a better stain than Freud did, and therefore visualized the structure more clearly.) Freud saw with his Hartnack No 10 microscope that dendrites terminate in the cell body – rather than 'pass through' it – and that axons likewise arise from the cell's cytoskeleton on the other side, thereby discovering that fibre and cell form a single unit.[1]

In addition, he sketched out the role of synaptic weighting in recording memories, two years before Sir Charles Sherrington even coined the term 'synapses' for the junctions between neurons, let alone articulated their fundamental role in memory formation. (Freud called them 'contact barriers': longer but clearer.)[2] The neurosurgeon and neuropsychologist Karl Pribram also acknowledged that Freud postulated that 'neurons that fire together wire together', more than 50 years before Donald Hebb said essentially the same thing.[3] So, Hebb's Law is really Freud's Law. And if we combine these two insights, all of a sudden we have the basic foundations for the neurophysiology of memory.

A similar story could be told about 'mirror neurons', which Giacomo Rizzolatti and Vittorio Gallese discovered in 1992, but whose functions Freud outlined in some detail almost 100 years earlier.[4] Gallese writes that 'the [Freudian] notions of projective identification and the interpersonal dynamic related to transference and countertransference can be viewed as instantiations of the implicit and prelinguistic mechanisms of the embodied simulation-driven mirroring mechanisms.'[5] This comment shows that Freud's early insights about the brain left a deep impression, not only on subsequent neuroscience, but also on his own basic concepts in psychoanalysis.

That's a brief synopsis of Freud's main contributions to neuroanatomy and neurophysiology. I could provide a similar list of his achievements in clinical neurology, and I have already indicated that he made foundational contributions to neuropsychology, though by attributing his contributions mainly to Luria perhaps I was insufficiently explicit about that. So, let me be clear: Luria's theory of 'dynamic localization' built directly upon Freud's much earlier critique of Broca-style localizationism in his *Conceptualizing the Aphasias* (1891).*

---

* The essential points that Freud made there were, first, that language is a psychological function the disorders of which must be analysed in *psychological* terms, not physiological ones. However, second, the complex functional system for language arises from an interaction between elementary component functions which *can* be anatomically localized. Therefore, third, the functional system for language (as Luria called it; Freud called it the 'language apparatus')

Contrary to Cobb's assertion, then, Freud's contributions to neuroscience, neurology and neuropsychology were both novel and insightful. Yet this was all just when he was explicitly and straightforwardly doing brain science. The true scale of his influence can only be appreciated when you get to grips with his later thought. Freud has had a huge – albeit concealed and sometimes disavowed – influence on our contemporary science of the brain, and he is still teaching us lots of important things about it.

In this chapter, I want to take stock of the contribution that *psychoanalysis* has made and still can make to neuroscience. I am going to concentrate upon what Freud brought to light about the functional organization of the brain as a whole, insofar as he was able to infer it from the phenomenology and organizing principles of our subjective mental life. We will see how modern neuroscience has taken up these Freudian ideas – often arriving at them independently, using different methods, which is one sort of vindication. At other times, it has simply followed in Freud's footsteps without realizing it. And sometimes it has been fully aware of its debt, yet chosen to hide it.

In setting out the main respects in which neuropsychology has arrived at Freudian conclusions, my purpose is not to settle scores. (Or not mainly that, anyway.) When we see how what Freud called 'the mental apparatus' fits together as a whole, and notice how well our modern conception of the mind now coincides with it, we may find that other aspects of his project start to make sense again, too. Psychoanalytic ideas can have extraordinary implications, which aren't always easily swallowed. We will explore some of these challenging propositions in later chapters. For now, let's start gently simmering the frog.

---

is something *virtual*. These three conclusions regarding language were generalizable to the mental apparatus as a whole. Thus, Freud the neurologist argued, just as Freud the psychoanalyst would later: 'psychical structures in general must never be regarded as localized in organic elements of the nervous system but rather, as one might say, *between* them' (Freud, 1900, p. 546). Any modern neuropsychologist will recognize this conceptualization as their own.

SUBJECTIVITY

Freud's first and biggest contribution to neuroscience was his recognition that science had hitherto neglected what is mental in its picture of the world:

> Psychoanalysis has a special right to speak for the scientific *Weltanschauung* [world view], since it cannot be reproached with having neglected what is mental in the picture of the world. Its contribution to science lies precisely in having extended research to the mental field. And, incidentally, without such a psychology science would be very incomplete.[6]

By 'mental' Freud didn't mean 'behavioural' or 'cognitive'. He meant 'subjective'. Science has always sought actively to exclude what is subjective from its view of the universe. That is why behaviourism declared subjective phenomena *data non grata*, and thereby excluded the psyche from psychology. For the same reason, Popper required that scientific theories must generate predictions which can be falsified objectively. That is all well and good, of course, except when it comes to understanding how and why subjectivity itself occurs. Without examining the peculiar characteristics of experience, including them in our picture of the world, we will never adequately understand the brain *or* the world. Accordingly, Oliver Sacks was moved to write:

> Neuropsychology, like classical neurology, aims to be entirely objective, and its great power, its advances, come from just this. But a living creature, and especially a human being, is first and last active – a subject, not an object. It is precisely the subject, the living 'I', which is being excluded. Neuropsychology is admirable, but it excludes the psyche – it excludes the experiencing, active, living 'I'.[7]

The philosopher David Chalmers asserted on a similar basis that neuropsychology – or cognitive neuroscience, as it has also come to be known* – addresses only the 'easy problem' of identifying the mechanisms that explain cognitive functions. In other words, it treats the brain like any other object. And yet, Chalmers points out, we can imagine a machine that, though devoid of experience, performs all the same objective functions as the brain. So how does experience itself arise? That's the hard problem.

> What makes the hard problem hard and almost unique is that it goes *beyond* problems about the performance of functions. To see this, note that even when we have explained the performance of all the cognitive and behavioural functions in the vicinity of experience [. . .] there may still remain a further unanswered question: *Why is the performance of these functions accompanied by experience?* A simple explanation of the functions leaves this question open [. . .] Why doesn't all this information processing go on 'in the dark', free of any inner feel?[8]

This gulf in cognitive neuroscience between mechanism and experience – what Chalmers and others call the 'explanatory gap' – led to the spooky conclusion that we need to add a new basic property to our physical conception of the universe. In other words, we need to add non-physical *mind stuff* to it. That means going all the way back to the dualism of Descartes, who proposed that reality itself was cleft into an objective, physical *res extensa* and a subjective, psychical *res cogitans*. Yet if mind isn't strictly speaking part of the world, then why does it seem so much as though it is *in* the world, acting on and responding to it? Dualists might be gesticulating from the other side, but the gap hasn't gone anywhere.

Unlike cognitive neuroscience, psychoanalysis *starts* from the fact that it feels like something to be a brain:

---

* I prefer 'neuropsychology', because 'cognitive neuroscience' excludes the psyche from its very name, which is what required Jaak Panksepp to develop an 'affective neuroscience'. Similar considerations led me to call the approach to neuropsychology that I advocate 'neuropsychoanalysis'.

> The starting point for this investigation is provided by a fact without parallel, which defies all explanation or description – the fact of consciousness. Nevertheless, if anyone speaks of consciousness we know immediately and from our most personal experience what is meant by it.[9]

Psychoanalysis accordingly takes as its subject matter the very thing that Sacks lamented was being excluded from neuropsychology: the experiencing, active, living 'I'.

The rupture between Freud's psychoanalytic research and his earlier work as a neuroscientist and neurologist occurred precisely here. What is not sufficiently appreciated is his justification for it: it was required, he said, not by any preference of his own, but by the nature of the subject. Unless we adjust our research methods to accommodate subjective experience, we shall never understand how the brain works.

We have seen what happened to our understanding of the causal mechanism of dreaming when we excluded the subjective side of the equation. Today, neuroscientists are far more willing to include subjective data. Yet it is important to distinguish Freud's reversal of the microscope from mere 'introspection', in the limited sense that it was used in the 19th century.[10] Freud's aim was to gather extensive samples of unedited *lived experience* obtained in a controlled setting. This required substantial personal commitment on the part of his research subjects, for which a precondition was a trusting relationship with him. The commitment was also facilitated greatly by clinical suffering: by the *need* to understand themselves.

On this basis, I and a small number of my co-workers have, since the 1990s, applied Freud's research method in clinical neuroscientific settings: systematically observing the effects upon lived experience of localized damage to different parts of the brain in neurological patients (and the effects of manipulations of different brain chemicals in psychiatric patients, and in normal controls). In other words, we have extended Freud and Luria's method to study the structure of personality, identifying its component functions through 'dynamic localization', just as Luria did with language, memory, attention and the like. There is no longer any good reason to exclude these chapters from our neuropsychological textbooks.

The research just mentioned provided new insights into the functional mechanisms of some neuropsychological disorders, such as Korsakoff syndrome and anosognosia,[11] and of some psychiatric disorders, such as major depression.[12] This shouldn't be surprising. What is it like to realize every minute or so that you do not have the foggiest clue what happened to you during the past few days, because you are suffering a dense amnesia, and will continue to suffer it for the rest of your life? Surely the *feeling* of this condition – and the things the feeling prompts you to do – will reveal something about the nature of the disorder, not to mention the function of remembering.

Freud's view was that subjectivity is just another part of nature. He gave a beautiful account of his approach, which I would like to quote at length:

> In our science as in others the problem is the same: behind the attributes (qualities) of the object under examination which are presented directly to our perception, we have to discover something else which is more independent of the particular receptive capacity of our sense organs and which approximates more closely to what may be supposed to be the real state of affairs. We have no hope of being able to reach the latter itself, since it is evident that everything new that we have inferred must nevertheless be translated back into the language of perceptions, from which it is simply impossible to free ourselves. But herein lies the very nature and limitation of our science. It is as though we were to say in physics: 'If we could see clearly enough we should find that what appears to be a solid body is made up of particles of such and such a shape and occupying such and such relative positions.' In the meantime, we try to increase the efficiency of our sense organs to the furthest possible extent by artificial aids; but it may be expected that all such efforts will fail to affect the ultimate outcome. Reality will

always remain 'unknowable' [. . .] Our procedure in psychoanalysis is quite similar. We have discovered technical methods of filling in the gaps in the phenomena of our consciousness, and we make use of those methods as a physicist makes use of experiments. In this manner we infer a number of processes which are in themselves 'unknowable' and interpolate them in those that are conscious to us. And if, for instance, we say: 'At this point an unconscious memory intervened', what that means is: 'At this point something occurred of which we are totally unable to form a conception, but which, if it had entered our consciousness, could only have been described in such and such a way.' Our justification for making such inferences and interpolations and the degree of certainty attaching to them of course remain open to criticism in each individual instance; and it cannot be denied that it is often extremely difficult to arrive at a decision – a fact which finds expression in the lack of agreement among analysts. The novelty of the problem is to blame for this – that is to say, a lack of training [. . .] But such sources of error, arising from the personal equation, have no great importance in the long run. If one looks through old textbooks on the use of the microscope, one is astonished to find the extraordinary demands which were made on the personality of those who made observations with the instrument while its technique was still young – of all of which there is no question today.[13]

Freud made no mention here of his own role in science's early efforts to discern the basic structure of the neuron using the microscope, so I will quote Shepherd:

The balanced judgement of Kölliker, the conceptual fixity of Golgi, the seething experimental and intellectual intensity of Cajal, the youthful energies of Nansen, the studious offerings of Freud – it is impossible not to be impressed by these personal qualities in studying their work.[14]

FUNCTIONALISM

Freud's response to the claim that there is an unbridgeable gap between the brain and subjective experience was that 'the brain' and 'subjective experience' are just two different perspectives upon one and the same thing. The brain that we see (in a brain scan, for example) is our perceptual experience of ourselves from the outside, as an object. The brain that we feel ourselves to be (with our eyes closed, for example) is our perceptual experience of ourselves from the inside, as a subject. What lies between these two classes of observable phenomena are the mechanisms that cause and explain them. This, on Freud's view, is the unifying object of study of *both* cognitive neuroscience and psychoanalysis:

> We know two kinds of things about what we call our psyche (or mental life): firstly, its bodily organ and scene of action, the brain (or nervous system) and, on the other hand, our acts of consciousness, which are immediate data and cannot be further explained by any sort of description. Everything that lies between is unknown to us [. . .] Our two hypotheses start from these ends or beginnings of our knowledge. The first is concerned with localization. We assume that mental life is the function of an apparatus to which we ascribe the characteristics of being extended in space and of being made up of several portions – which we imagine, that is, as resembling a telescope or microscope or something of the kind. Notwithstanding some earlier attempts in the same direction, the consistent working out of a conception such as this is a scientific novelty.[15]

Despite Cobb's claim, the 'scientific novelty' that Freud introduced here (in 1900) is the standard approach in cognitive neuroscience today. It's called *functionalism*.* Freud called it 'dissecting the function'. He added: 'So far as I know, the experiment has not

---

* There are many different kinds of 'functionalism'. I am referring here to functionalism as a philosophy of mind.

hitherto been made of using this method of dissection in order to investigate the way in which the mental instrument is put together, and I can see no harm in it [...] so long as we retain the coolness of our judgement and do not mistake the scaffolding for the building'.[16]

The basic idea was this: what defines and explains the mind is what the brain *does*, not the material that it uses to do it.* We infer its underlying functions from the data of perception (whether they be objective or subjective). Thus, we speak of abstracted entities like 'memory systems', which we infer from both the material phenomenology of neural traces *and* the psychical phenomenology of felt reminiscences. Nowadays, we describe the underlying functioning of the memory systems themselves in terms of information processing. Information is physical, in the sense of physics, but we cannot see it with our eyes; we *infer* it from its physiological and psychological effects.

Functionalism, as a philosophy of mind, is generally attributed not to Freud (1900) but rather to Hilary Putnam, and dated to the 1960s. There are philosophical grounds on which you might reject it, as indeed there are for any part of science and the whole of it. It has some troubling implications, which we shall discuss later. Be that as it may, the set of abstracted functional systems that Freud called the 'mental apparatus' just is the ultimate object of study of psychoanalysts *and* of cognitive neuroscientists; and the functionalist approach itself was a conceptual innovation of Freud's.

---

* Freud (1926, pp. 172–3) writes: 'It will soon be clear what the mental apparatus is; but I must beg you not to ask what material it is constructed of. That is not a subject of psychological interest. Psychology can be as indifferent to it as, for instance, optics can be to the question of whether the walls of the telescope are made of metal or cardboard. We shall leave entirely on one side the *material* line of approach, but not so the *spatial* one. For we picture the unknown apparatus which serves the activities of the mind as really being an instrument constructed of several parts (which we speak of as "agencies") [today, we speak of "systems" or "modules"], each of which performs a particular *function* and which have a fixed spatial relation to each other.'

Functionalism is not only an ontological position (what is the mind made of?). It is also an epistemological strategy (how can we understand it?). If the brain is indeed the most complicated thing in the known universe, whose synaptic connections outnumber the stars in the sky and so on, what would it take to fathom such a thing?

The functionalist approach is to zoom out from the minutiae of what goes on at the level of each neuron (or each free association) and attempt to abstract the general principles governing the overall patterns. If we do this from both ends of the microscope, we can reasonably hope that our inferences might meet somewhere in the middle. This is what Freud hoped we would achieve when he first coined the term 'metapsychology': he wanted to 'transform metaphysics into metapsychology'.[17] In other words, he wanted to replace philosophical speculation about the mind/body relation with a scientific strategy that bridged the gap between its two phenomenological manifestations. He asked us not to judge too harshly his initial descriptions of what lies between them, couched in provisional, stopgap terms such as 'memory systems' and 'drives':

> This is merely due to our being obliged to operate with the scientific terms, that is to say with the figurative language, peculiar to psychology (or, more precisely, to depth psychology). We could not otherwise describe the processes in question at all, and indeed we could not even become aware of them. The deficiencies in our description would probably vanish if we were already in a position to replace the psychological terms by physiological and chemical ones.[18]

The last sentence is crucial. It *must* be possible to describe things like 'memory systems' and 'drives' both psychologically and physiologically; but in Freud's day, we lacked the technical resources to tackle the physiological side of the equation.

THE UNCONSCIOUS

Like Darwin in relation to the multiplicity of biological species, Freud was not content to merely describe and classify mental phenomena; he sought to *explain* them. But here he encountered a puzzle. The mental world that we can access from the subjective point of view turns out to be full of missing links: strange jumps and elisions moving between topics and judgements as if along chains of hidden premises. One second you're wondering what to have for lunch, the next you're googling 'gluten intolerant rodents'. What marvellous hidden infrastructure conveys you from A to B at such speed?

When Freud was developing his explanations, *conscious* thinking was believed to be the only thinking there was, by definition.* Thus, for example, Franz Brentano, the professor of philosophy at the University of Vienna when Freud was a student there, wrote: 'The question, "Is there unconscious consciousness?"† is to be answered with a firm, "No".'[19]

Something had to give. Either your conscious thought is complete but nonsensical, or some of your thoughts must be unconscious. Freud couldn't accept the former conclusion, so he took the inevitable step:

> Conscious processes do not form unbroken sequences which are complete in themselves; there would thus be no alternative left to assuming that there are physical or somatic processes which are concomitant with the psychical ones and which we should necessarily have to recognize as more complete than the psychical sequences, since some of them would have conscious processes parallel to them but others would not.

---

* This is not to deny that many people before Freud spoke of unconscious processes in a physiological, psychophysical, philosophical and even mystical sense.

† The strange term 'unconscious *consciousness*' must be understood in historical context: it meant 'unconscious *mind*'.

> If so, it of course becomes plausible to lay stress in psychology on these somatic processes, to see in *them* the true essence of what is psychical and to look for some other assessment of the conscious processes. The majority of philosophers, however, as well as many other people, dispute this and declare that the idea of something psychical being unconscious is self-contradictory. But that is precisely what psychoanalysis is obliged to assert [. . .] It explains the supposedly somatic concomitant phenomena as being what is truly psychical.[20]

Freud's reasoning here was subtle, and therefore easily misunderstood. He wanted to know why, if the brain and the mind are two observational perspectives upon one and the same thing, our external perception of that thing seems to be more complete than our internal perception of it. His answer was: the internal perspective must include both conscious and unconscious parts; there must be both conscious *and unconscious* thoughts, memories, beliefs, and so forth.

Unlike functionalism, which might be described as a fruitful conceptual framework, Freud's inference that there is such a thing as unconscious mental processes was a genuine *discovery*, though it took cognitive science eighty years to catch up to him. It is true that cognitive neuroscientists did not simply adopt his views; they rediscovered unconscious mental processes independently, using many different methods. Nevertheless, neuroscience clearly owes Freud credit on this score.

What is more, I don't think that most cognitive neuroscientists have yet fully appreciated the implications of the fact that conscious psychological processes are caused by unconscious *psychological* processes (which can also be *viewed* as physiological processes). As Freud wrote, there is no reason to assume that they can be understood best from a physiological perspective, rather than by adapting our models of thinking to the peculiarities of how thinking behaves when there is no one around to watch it. He elaborated:

It is possible to establish the laws which they [conscious and unconscious thoughts] obey and to follow their mutual relations and interdependencies unbroken over long stretches – in short to arrive at what is called an 'understanding' of the field of natural phenomena in question. This cannot be effected without framing fresh hypotheses and creating fresh concepts; but these are not to be despised as evidence of embarrassment on our part but deserve on the contrary to be appreciated as an enrichment of science. They can lay claim to the same value as approximations that belong to the corresponding intellectual scaffolding found in other natural sciences, and we look forward to them being modified, corrected and more precisely determined as further experience is accumulated and sifted.[21]

And one of the most important among the fresh concepts (or approximations) that Freud introduced was that of drives.

DRIVES

Despite impressive competition, 'libido' might be the most misunderstood term in classical psychoanalytic jargon. The fact that in popular usage it means simply 'sexual appetite' can't really be held against popular usage, since, as we shall see later, Freud himself was both vague and indecisive about the extent to which all appetites are sexual. Yet, even if we use the less compromised term 'drive energy', this remains an enigmatic concept.

From the moment that he made the transition from brain science to psychoanalysis, Freud insisted that the 'higher' functions studied by psychology and neuropsychology could only have evolved to serve the 'lower' biological needs of the organism. Whatever else we human beings are, *Homo sapiens* is a species of animal. (Even this contention brought Freud notoriety in Victorian times.)

So, how many innate needs does the human animal have, actually? Strangely enough, Freud sometimes seemed to think that the answer was: *one*. The singular need in question was the pursuit of pleasure (and avoidance of unpleasure).* Freud observed that we are motivated by pleasure for its own sake, independently of its survival value. Thus, babies suckle at the breast even when they aren't hungry, simply because they like it; likewise, people eat chocolate because it tastes good, not because it augments their glucose supplies. And, of course, people frequently engage in sexual acts when they aren't trying to procreate – and some plainly sexual acts can't possibly result in babies. For all these reasons, and more, Freud grappled with the idea that the pursuit of any pleasure for its own sake should be described as 'sexual'.

As choices of umbrella category go, this one seems particularly questionable. So, for decades, Freud's notion of a single fungible essence that powers and explains purposive action – 'the *mainspring* of the psychical mechanism'[22] – has baffled his admirers (both researchers and clinicians alike) while lending ammunition to those who accuse him of pseudoscience, or worse.

Nevertheless, since the 1990s, Freud's odd conjecture has become central to one of the most promising areas in theoretical neuroscience. Rather astonishingly, the cranky philosophical notion of a universal drive, variously construed as libido, Wilhelm Reich's 'orgone', Henri Bergson's *élan vital*, the Hobbesian drive for self-preservation, Schopenhauer's will to live, Nietzsche's will to power and so on, now has a precise mathematical expression. In its new form, it sheds light not only on the workings of the mind but also on the basic thermodynamic constraints acting on all self-organizing entities, and therefore on the origin of life and mind.†

---

* Freud took the view that the satisfaction of self-preservative needs (like hunger and thirst) is pleasurable only secondarily, by dint of an 'anaclitic' association with sexuality. On this basis, he eventually combined the sexual and self-preservative drives under the single heading of 'life drives', which he contrasted with a 'death drive'. At that point, he concluded that we pursue not only pleasure but also *quiescence* (see Chapter Five).

† In a slightly extended sense, it underlies the mathematics of some deep algorithms that power the current artificial intelligence boom. (See Parr, Pezzulo & Friston, 2022.)

Freud defined a psychological version of the concept, quite serviceably, as follows:

> 'Drive' appears to us as a [. . .] psychical representative of the stimuli originating from within the organism and reaching the mind, as *a measure of the demand made upon the mind for work* in consequence of its connection with the body.[23]

The psychoanalyst and psychiatrist Mortimer Ostow was the first to point out that this bore a striking resemblance to the concept of 'free energy', originally a measure of the thermodynamic efficiency of steam engines. In 1962, he wrote of Freud's notion that all mental work seemed to pursue a single ultimate end:

> It is reasonable to compare it to the behaviour of thermodynamic free energy which creates the impression of an inherent 'striving' to discharge itself [. . .] When he spoke of 'psychic energy' and libido, Freud conceived of an entity *analogous* to thermodynamic free energy, an analogy he often extended to contrasting 'bound energy' with 'free energy'.[24]

In my experience, people find this an intensely alien notion the first time they hear it, but after toying with it for a while, it can become intuitive. I'll try to help you speed-run that process, but don't worry if it still sounds like nonsense by the end of this section: it's not an essential part of the argument of this book.

Here's one way of thinking about it. A steam engine is a physical structure that burns fuel to boil water, turning it into steam. The steam then flows at pressure into the cylinder of a piston or past a wheel to drive a mechanism that does useful work. Through incremental refinements to the design of such a device, you can keep increasing the amount of work you get in exchange for each unit of power. You can make sure that there are no leaks, that the wheel turns freely, that the channel along which the steam flows is as short and well-insulated as possible so that it doesn't dissipate heat, cool down and lose pressure on its journey, and so on. Perfect efficiency is impossible, but as a guiding ideal it is very clear what efficiency asks of steam-engine design: each mechanism must 'bind' as much energy as possible in the service of its desired outputs. Bound energy is good; free energy is a problem.

A living body is also a physical structure. It uses the data that flows in through its senses to decide what, if anything, will need to change if it is to stay alive and healthy. Changing things is thermodynamically expensive: small changes take effort and big ones take innumerable deaths over aeons of evolutionary time. Ideally, then, everything will be able to stay more or less as it is. This means that, ideally, the data flowing in through the body's senses will have been anticipated in advance. Predicted data flows harmlessly through the system demanding no alterations: it is like the 'bound' portion of the heat energy flowing through a steam engine that helps to drive the piston. Unpredicted data, on the other hand, is a problem: *something* is out there that we didn't expect, and so something will need to change – but what? It's like the 'free' portion of the heat energy that the engine wastes, or that wastes the engine, accelerating its disintegration through wear and tear.

Perfect predictive efficiency is, of course, impossible. Yet as a guiding ideal it is very clear what it asks, of biological evolution and individual development alike: organisms that correctly and frugally anticipate as much of what happens to them as possible, in the service of survival and reproduction. Bound energy is good: it means that the inner structures of the organism fit the relevant features of its environment, allowing it to avoid threats and take advantage of opportunities. Free energy is a problem: the senses bring news that all is not as expected, and so the randomness of the exterior threatens to penetrate the order of the citadel. Since self-sustaining order is the essence of every living being, minimizing free energy through continual improvements in predictive efficiency must in some sense be the master objective of life itself: it is what shapes organisms at every level of organization, from organelles to organigrams.

Karl Friston was the one who recognized that, while the drive to exist against a backdrop of cosmic entropy does indeed impose hard thermodynamic constraints, the actual free energy at work in the mind is not thermodynamic but *informational*. It is a measure of the brain's level of uncertainty, in both the statistical and psychological sense, as it tries to work out how to meet its biological needs. Thanks to Claude Shannon's invention of information theory in the 1940s, it is now possible to quantify information in much the same way as we quantify thermodynamic energy, and with very similar mathematics. This allowed Friston, via his Free Energy Principle and closely related 'active inference' framework in computational neuroscience, to achieve what Freud only dreamed of: the representation of mental processes as relationships between quantities.* With this piece of the puzzle in place, it would be hard to state the role of free energy in the mind better than Freud did himself: it is precisely 'a measure of the demand made upon the mind for work in consequence of its connection with the body.'

This framework is now being used to tackle many longstanding puzzles in neuroscience, psychology and psychiatry, ranging from the unity of perception and action to the causes of 'functional neurological disorders' and false beliefs – and even to the nature of subjectivity, the solution of the mind/body problem, and the origin of life. Friston explicitly notes the equivalence of his version of the free energy concept and Freud's 'drive energy', and their common roots in the 19th-century physics and physiology of Hermann von Helmholtz.[25]

Still, while Friston is the most cited neuroscientist in the world today, his framework is not hegemonic. That being so, perhaps we should chalk up Freud's notion of drive energy as one of the most promising intuitions he had, rather than one that has already

---

* It is important to note that the free energy of complex organisms is not a continuous variable only; it is distributed over a number of categorical variables. Our multiple needs cannot be reduced to a common denominator. And so our drives must be *qualitatively* distinctive: 8/10 of sleepiness is not the same as 8/10 of thirst. This is perhaps the natural origin of what philosophers call 'qualia': the distinctively different feelings of different feelings.

achieved universal consensus in the mental sciences.* There's everything still to play for.

WISHFULNESS

This leads us to the next of Freud's major contributions to neuroscience: his realization that cognition is, at bottom, *wishful*. You might have encountered the notion that the brain is a 'prediction machine', popularised by Anil Seth (2021a), Andy Clark (2015) and many others. In modern neuroscience, we know that when our biological needs press upon us, they elicit various plans and suggestions about what we should do to reduce them (that is, to 'bind' the free energy and keep us out of trouble).

Where do these intentions – in effect, predictions about what will work – come from? Well, firstly, from inborn instinct (i.e., from natural selection), and later, from what we learn through experience. We must supplement our instincts through learning, because the instincts alone are too crudely stereotyped to meet our needs in all contexts. So, learning happens when we save for future use an action that experience has taught us will bring about the desired outcome. Almost a century before predictive processing began to dominate theoretical neuroscience, this is exactly how Freud formulated it in *The Interpretation of Dreams*:

> The exigencies of life confront us first in the form of the major somatic needs. The excitations produced by internal needs seek discharge in movement, which may be described as an 'internal change' or an 'expression of emotion'. A hungry baby screams or kicks helplessly. But the situation remains unaltered [. . .] A change can only come about if in some way or other

---

* This is not the place to convey the profundity and richness of the Free Energy Principle. For interested readers wanting a digestible introduction, I recommend Jakob Hohwy's *The Predictive Mind* (2013). For a possibly less digestible treatment, I recommend my own *The Hidden Spring* (2021).

(in the case of the baby, through outside help) an 'experience of satisfaction' can be achieved which puts an end to the internal stimulus. An essential component of this experience of satisfaction is a particular perception (that of nourishment, in our example) the memory image of which remains associated thenceforward with the memory trace of the excitation produced by the need. As a result of the link that has thus been established, next time this need arises a mental impulse will at once emerge which will seek to re-activate the memory image of the perception and to re-evoke the perception itself, that is to say, to re-establish the situation of the original satisfaction. An impulse of this kind is what we call a wish; the re-appearance of the perception is the fulfilment of the wish; and the shortest path to the fulfilment of a wish is a path leading directly from the excitation produced by the need to a complete activation of the perception.[26]

Today we might rephrase Freud's last sentence like this: An impulse of this kind is what we call a *prediction*; the re-appearance of the perception is the *confirmation of the prediction*. Karl Friston made this point in an article for the influential journal *Trends in Cognitive Science*, under the uncompromisingly Freudian title 'All Thinking is "Wishful" Thinking' (2020).[27]

But there is more. The above quotation from Freud continues as follows:

Nothing prevents us from assuming that there was a primitive state of the mental apparatus in which this path was actually traversed, that is, in which *wishing ended in hallucinating*. Thus, the aim of this first psychical activity was to produce a 'perceptual identity' – a repetition of the perception which was linked with the satisfaction of the need.[28]

To be clear: Freud is claiming that there may have been a time when prediction (wishing) naturally ended in hallucination. This was considered unlikely when he first published it in 1900, and understandably so. In neuroscience today, however, the notion that perception occurs through 'controlled hallucination' is widely accepted.

The emphasis falls on the word 'controlled'. Wishful thinking needs to be tempered by some capacity to acknowledge and adjust when it goes wrong. Freud called this aspect of cognition 'reality testing', and it formed the basis of what he called the 'secondary process'. The above quotation continues:

> The bitter experience of life must have changed this primitive thought activity into a more expedient secondary one. The establishment of a perceptual identity along the short path of regression* within the apparatus does not have the same result elsewhere in the mind as does the same perception from without. Satisfaction does not follow; the need persists [. . .] In order to arrive at a more efficient expenditure of psychical energy, it is necessary to bring the regression to a halt before it becomes complete, so that it does not proceed beyond the memory image [to perception and therefore hallucination], and is able to seek out other paths which lead eventually to the desired perceptual identity being established from the direction of the external world. This inhibition of regression and the subsequent diversion of the excitation become the business of a second system, which is in control of voluntary movement.[29]

In other words: the fulfilment of our wishes through hallucination alone doesn't satisfy our real biological needs. In order to save mental energy (to be the most efficient engines we can be), we must stop the hallucination before it comes up short, and instead divert our mental efforts toward actions that might really bring about the desired 'perceptual identity': that is, sensory confirmation that our

---

* This term refers to mental functions – like dreaming – which proceed backwards from the memory systems on to the perceptual system (see Figure 2, p. 114). 'Progressive' mental functions, by contrast, proceed in the forward direction, towards the motor system.

need has been satisfied in reality and not only in our imaginations. I hope it is clear just how prescient this formulation was. Compare it to a contemporary version by Anil Seth:

> We're all hallucinating all the time. Every perception we have is an act of construction, an act of interpretation in which the brain's expectations about what's out there in the world are reined in, or controlled by, sensory signals coming from the world. I like to think of perception as controlled hallucination. It's a construction, but it is controlled by what's out there in the world. What we typically call hallucination, when people see things that other people don't, we can think of as a form of *uncontrolled* perception in which the brain's predictions are *not* being reined in by what's out there in the world.[30]

Neuroscientists who say things like this almost never cite Freud. Even so, it's clear that our modern understanding of how the brain works has become very notably Freudian in this respect.

By the way, Freud thought that the sleeping mind lacks the inhibitory 'secondary process' he just described. It lacks 'reality testing' (which we now call 'prediction error'), precisely because it has withdrawn from reality into the state of sleep. That is why dreams take the form of hallucinatory wish-fulfilments. The quotation from Freud, above, ends as follows:

> Dreams, which fulfil their wishes along the short path of regression, have merely preserved for us in that respect a sample of the psychical apparatus's primary method of working, a method which was abandoned as being inefficient.[31]

What is the standing of this formulation of dreaming in modern neuroscience? Well, let me just say that Allan Hobson, the neurophysiologist who claimed to have disproven Freudian dream theory before I in turn disproved his theory, ultimately teamed up with Karl Friston; and they concluded exactly as Freud did in the passage just quoted, namely that dreaming is the primary form of consciousness: 'Dream consciousness and its physiological underpinnings [are] a virtual reality model of the world that prepares us for waking consciousness.'[32] Hobson called it 'protoconsciousness'.

FEELINGS

I said earlier that whatever else we human beings are, *Homo sapiens* is a species of animal. But how did human *being* come about? Why is there 'something it is like' to be a human organism?

Freud's answer started from his concept of drive. He observed that the human infant is born with a set of innate needs. These needs arise from the fact that we human beings, like all living things, must remain within our biologically viable bounds. This is uncontroversial, the most basic of all biological principles. What is distinctively 'Freudian' about the claim, then, is not the brute existence of innate needs, but rather their implications for the life of the mind.

We have already quoted Freud's assertion that our biological drives are 'the mainspring of the psychical mechanism'. By this he meant that they are literally what brings subjective being into being. On his view, they do this because they are consciously felt: drive demand is *unpleasant* and drive satisfaction is *pleasant*. Freud called this the 'pleasure principle'. Modern neuroscientists such as Antonio Damasio[33] call it an extended form of 'homeostasis': increasing deviation from our biologically viable bounds (from homeostatic 'set-points') is felt as unpleasure, and returning toward the set-points is felt as pleasure. According to Damasio, this is why feeling evolved: feeling enables organisms to know whether they are increasing or decreasing their chances of survival, before it's too late. So, feeling is the basis of *choice*.

And then we can learn from our felt experiences. In behaviourist times, this basic mechanism of learning was called the Law of Effect:

Responses that produce a rewarding effect in a particular situation become more likely to occur again in that situation, and responses that produce a punishing effect become less likely to occur again in that situation.[34]

The behaviourist school in psychology didn't think this had anything to do with feelings. They thought it was a basic law of *behaviour*. 'Rewards' and 'punishments' were not considered to be subjective events; they were construed as objective 'stimuli' which elicited objective 'responses'. As far as they were concerned, such functions might very well be going on in the dark. Indeed, from a behaviourist perspective, the distinction between a conscious being and an automaton collapses altogether. That is what is at stake here: the very existence of the mind.

As a dualist, the philosopher David Chalmers can hardly be accused of denying the mind's existence. Even so, he seems to overlook it just when it matters most. When he wrote that 'there is no cognitive function such that we can say in advance that explanation of that function will automatically explain experience', he implies that neuroscience is limited to explaining *cognition*.[35] Thinking, learning, remembering, planning – all of these cognitive functions can indeed go on in the dark, as Freud was the first to point out. Yet it is clear that an explanation of the function of *feeling* will automatically explain experience. If you don't explain why feelings feel like something, you haven't explained them. Feeling requires consciousness. There can be no such thing as feelings that you don't feel.

It doesn't matter that Freud knew next to nothing about homeostasis,[36] or that he called the Law of Effect the 'pleasure principle', or that he assigned this mode of mental functioning to a metapsychological abstraction called 'the id' (a term that nobody outside of psychoanalysis uses anymore). It also doesn't matter that Freud's pioneering attempts at classifying the drives were hopelessly wrong (in fairness, he predicted in 1920 that the biology of the future would 'blow away' his speculations in this regard).[37] It turns out that there are many varieties of pleasure in the brain, modulated by many different chemicals, only a few of which may reasonably be regarded as sexual. These details are neither here nor there; what matters is Freud's foundational premise that the mind is *driven* and that it is literally constituted by its capacity for feeling how well or badly it is satisfying its drives.

Neuroscience has moved on from Freud, identifying brain circuits that link a variety of innate needs to what appear to be distinct primary feelings, not reducible to each other. But it is still working within a basically Freudian conception of what feeling *is*. And while Freud's mistakes regarding the details have not been without theoretical and therapeutic ill-effects over the years, a basically Freudian model of drives and feelings, combined with a basically Freudian model of how memory and learning work, fine-tuned a little by cognitive neuroscience (as we shall see now), may be our best hope for treating emotional disorders (as we shall see next).

MULTIPLE MEMORY SYSTEMS

In 1896 Freud wrote to his friend, Wilhelm Fliess:*

> What is essentially new about my theory is the thesis that memory is present not once but several times over, that it is laid down in various kinds of indications. [. . .] I cannot say how many of these registrations there are: at least three, probably more.[38]

---

* Fliess was an otolaryngologist who lived and worked in Berlin. He was also a bit of a crank. He developed a properly pseudoscientific theory about human biorhythms, and he proposed physiological connections between the nose and the genitals that simply don't exist. Today he is best remembered for his close friendship with Freud, for whom he acted as a sounding board while he was developing his earliest theories – so much so that Google erroneously lists him under the heading 'German psychoanalyst'. What Freud saw in him remains a topic of scholarly debate.

How extraordinary that Freud could infer this almost entirely from psychoanalytical observations – that is, from talking to his patients and looking within himself. Memory is indeed present not once but several times over, and it is indeed laid down in various different kinds of neurophysiological registrations.

Even more impressive, Freud worked out that there must be at least *three* main types of registration: what he termed 'conscious' (now called short-term memory), 'preconscious' (declarative long-term memory) and 'unconscious' (nondeclarative long-term memory). The fundamental difference between declarative and nondeclarative long-term memory is that the former type of memory can be retrieved into (conscious) short-term memory, whereas the latter type cannot; this is exactly the distinction that Freud drew between his preconscious and unconscious systems. And it is just this distinction that gave his 'depth psychology' the dimension of depth. Today, the 'multiple memory systems' model is the standard model used in all of neuropsychology. Once again, Freud is not given credit, and to add insult to injury, the idea is conventionally attributed to Edward Tolman (1948) – a behaviourist.

Though arguably implicit in the very idea of multiple systems, it's notable how clearly Freud saw that memories must be able to move from one system to another in an ongoing, active process. As he wrote to Fliess in the same letter:

> I am working on the assumption that our psychical mechanism has come into being by a process of stratification: the material present in the form of memory traces being subjected from time to time to a *rearrangement* in accordance with fresh circumstances – to a *retranscription*.

We now call these processes 'systems consolidation' and 'reconsolidation', both of which were rediscovered completely independently of Freud, using different methods. The fact that memory encoding involves an ongoing process of consolidation was inferred from the finding that recent memories are wiped out *retroactively* — the oldest ones being the most stable – following brain injury. That there are multiple memory systems was inferred from the finding that damage to different parts of the brain leads to dissociations between different categories of memory.

The most important such dissociation was the finding that patients who are unable to encode new *declarative* long-term memories are nevertheless capable of learning *unconsciously*. (This is one of the ways in which the unconscious returned to neuroscience.) Reconsolidation was rediscovered in the early 21st century, through a finding that long-term memories are wiped out if protein synthesis is inhibited when they are returned to the short-term state. (Since protein synthesis is required for the formation of new long-term memories, this demonstrates that our declarative memories are literally dissolved and then encoded afresh each time they are retrieved.)

Isn't the fact that Freud was able to intuit the broad outline of all this, merely by listening closely to what his patients told him, just astounding? Even now, it pretty well knocks me off my feet every time I stop to think about it.

Reconsolidation is important because it is the fundamental mechanism by which our errors can update our predictive models. This occurs when an expected event fails to materialize, resulting in a state of uncertainty. Since this has been a preoccupation of my own recent scientific work, I hope you will forgive a touch of partisanship when I propose that contemporary cognitive neuroscience has neglected the link between this surge of uncertainty and the ultimate function of consciousness. What, after all, is our inner light of consciousness *for*? Unless evolution dropped the ball in quite an uncharacteristic way, the answer presumably has something to do with what it actually *does*.

Everyone is familiar with how, when things don't work out as expected, we become sharply alert to our surroundings. Think how it feels on a long, lulling journey when you miss your turning: you leave autopilot mode and scramble to reconcile where you are with where you should be. A colloquial term for this kind of experience is *wake-up call*: it literally summons consciousness to sort things out and make the necessary adjustments, inside and out, so that you can sleepwalk the entire way undisturbed next time.

In such situations, Freud observed (in another connection), 'consciousness arises instead of a memory trace'.[39] We look lively, we pay attention, we depart from the script. Long-term memories are rendered labile in the process of reconsolidation by a part of the upper brainstem called the reticular activating system. This is the part of the brain that wakes you up in the morning and puts you to sleep at night. (Damage there results in coma.) It squirts chemical neuromodulators up into the region of the forebrain that stored the memory (the prediction) that was supposed to get you home. Mightn't this odd piece of neurophysiological engineering have something to tell us about the workings of consciousness more generally? If so, Freud's contribution to modern neuroscience might not be finished yet.

By the way, while I am sharing hunches, it surely can't be an accident that dreaming is a *conscious* state. In my view, consciousness intrudes during sleep because incongruities between memory traces come to light during the consolidation process that certainly occurs while our minds are offline. The mental work of dreaming would therefore be an attempt to reconcile newly acquired memories (products of the day's prediction errors) with existing predictions. Since the most heartfelt beliefs are not relinquished easily, this would at a stroke account both for the wishfulness of dreams and for some of their weirdness.

Whatever the empirical fate of this speculation, I hope it is clear that Freud's conjecture about the existence of multiple memory systems has been triumphantly fruitful for modern neuroscience.

CRITICAL PERIODS

The 'process of stratification' that Freud noticed in our memories includes a recent discovery that would have pleased him enormously: the declarative long-term memory systems kick in only during the third year of life.⁴⁰ This accounts for much of what he called 'infantile amnesia'.

Today we speak about a more general phenomenon called 'critical periods'. These are stages in life when the nervous system is especially sensitive to specific environmental stimuli. During such phases, the brain is much better at certain types of learning. A well-known example is the window for easy language acquisition; once a critical period ends, the relevant skill or attribute becomes far harder to develop. Happily, the same applies the other way around: the brain is relatively immune to some noxious events if they occur *prior* to a critical period. For example, if the left hemisphere is surgically removed in pre-verbal infancy (for the control of severe epilepsy arising from damage to that hemisphere), the right hemisphere develops all the language and other functions that would normally have been assigned to the left.

The general version of the concept was first named by Charles Stockard in the 1920s, yet Freud clearly got close to the same insight in the 1890s. He called them dispositional fixation points. I will skip over the details here, because he got many of them wrong, but this is a statement of the general idea:

> In my search for the pathogenic situations [. . .] I was carried further and further back into the patient's life and ended by reaching the first years of his childhood. What poets and students of human nature had always asserted turned out to be true: the impressions of that remote period of life, though they were for the most part buried in amnesia, left ineradicable traces upon the individual's development.⁴¹

Languages and skills aren't the only things we can pick up during periods of peculiar receptiveness, of course, under the cover of peculiar forgetfulness. Some pretty important memories are laid down in the first two years of your life, too, and they can only be laid down in nondeclarative unconscious form. Attachment bonding, for example, occurs during the first six months, and this really does result in 'ineradicable traces', for good or ill. Much of the drama of psychoanalytic therapy consists precisely in trying to reconstruct from indirect evidence what happened in these developmental blind spots.

Freud's *oeuvre* contains many items that seem to defy the reader to ask: is he having me on? One such oddity is his speculative psychobiography of the 15th-century polymath, Leonardo da Vinci. A prominent part in Freud's study is played by Leonardo's 'memory' of being visited in his cradle by a bird of prey which stuck its tail into his mouth; Freud doubted the veracity of this recollection and interpreted it instead as a retrospective fantasy of fellatio. Yet it is this study that gave rise to one of the rare occasions when a notable modern neuroscientist acknowledged the pathfinding value of Freud's work. As the eminent visual scientist Semir Zeki said:*

> Neurobiologists may well raise an eyebrow at the quality of Freud's evidence; they may be appalled by his retrospective approach. But none can deny the seriousness with which he approached the subject or, in the context of what we have since learned, the physiological basis of his conclusions.[42]

The crux of Freud's analysis was that Leonardo's father disowned him at birth, only reuniting with him when he was five years old: 'And by then it was too late. In the first three or four years of life certain impressions become fixed and ways of reacting to the outside world are established which can *never* be deprived of their importance by later experiences.'[43] Zeki comments:

---

* Zeki is a Fellow of the Royal Society and was editor of the *Philosophical Transactions of the Royal Society* (B) from 1997 to 2004. He made fundamental contributions to our understanding of the brain mechanisms for colour vision. In view of the earlier discussion of 'controlled hallucination', it is instructive to note that Zeki recognized as early as 1993 that colour doesn't exist – as such, as colour – in the outside world; it is '*a property of the brain*, a property with which it invests the surfaces outside, an interpretation it gives to certain physical properties of objects' (Zeki, 1993, p. 236; emphasis added).

> Freud sought to dissect out the various influences that may operate in early childhood in establishing the later personality of the individual. To most neurobiologists this is too daunting a task, because it deals with so many unknowns and so many variables [. . .] Yet Freud's approach has been refined in stages, from specific kinds of complex behaviour right down to the development of specific pathways and the responses of single cells in the cortex. And in general terms the conclusions that Freud reached from studying complex behaviour have been found to be mirrored at the single cell level.[44]

In this regard, Zeki cites the research of the famous ethologist Harry Harlow, which demonstrated experimentally the importance for mental development of early maternal contact. In the late 1950s, Harlow separated infant rhesus monkeys from their mothers and raised them in cages in a laboratory setting. Their bodily needs (such as for food and water) were met, but they were deprived of emotional contact. These isolated monkeys behaved in a disturbed fashion, staring blankly, circling their cages, and mutilating themselves. It was impossible to rehabilitate them. Harlow concluded that 'there is a critical period somewhere between the third and sixth months of life during which social deprivation [. . .] irreversibly blights the animal's capacity for social adjustment.'[45] Similar phenomena were observed, later, in human beings who were raised in Romanian orphanages during the Soviet era. Zeki comments:

> The experimental approach, the ability to study the development of personality *forward* in time enabled Harlow to be more precise about the critical period than Freud had been able to from his retrospective approach, but the conclusions were the same.[46]

Freud's role in identifying the special formative power of infantile experiences has received something like its due in the modern psychological literature. (It helps that Harlow was strongly influenced by the psychoanalyst John Bowlby, and that he later became an outspoken Freudian himself.) But what a fertile theme it has been, for neuroscience in particular.

The research of Michael Meaney, with whom I worked briefly at the Hope for Depression Research Foundation, is especially interesting here. Meaney demonstrated that rat pups deprived of early maternal contact show abnormally high stress responses, for life, and that these responses are related to specific structural brain changes.* Remarkably, the changes are determined by *gene expression*. Meaney therefore established a causal relationship between maternal care and the selection of certain epigenetic programmes: a switch between modes of physical growth and development, triggered in infancy, that remain engaged for the entire life of the animal.

He also studied the relationship between maternal care and epigenetic programming in oestrogen receptor expression in the brain. His results showed that rat pups deprived of early maternal care grow up to be uncaring mothers themselves, even if, following the critical period of deprivation, they were fostered to high-caring mothers.

This is a sobering result. Rats and humans differ in lots of obvious ways, but generally speaking, the critical impact of early experience is even more decisive in human beings than it is in other species. To facilitate the passage of our large heads through the birth canal, we are born with less mature brains than any other animal. This means that we have a greater degree and longer period of dependency, so the early caregiving environment has an even larger impact upon our mental health. In Meaney's experiments, we glimpse a possible epigenetic explanation for the ways in which patterns of care or neglect often repeat themselves down through the generations – unless we can find ways to break the cycle.

---

* Viz., glucocorticoid receptor density in the hypothalamic-pituitary-adrenal axis.

What does Freud's theoretical contribution to modern neuroscience amount to? There are of course areas of controversy in cognitive and affective neuroscience, just as there are in any empirical discipline. Yet it is fair to say that our state-of-the-art conceptions of the nature and function of consciousness, the centrality of feeling and emotion, the embodied roots of cognition, the subjectively constructed and predictive nature of perception, the dimension of depth in our multiple memory systems, the astonishing degree to which our thinking and behaviour are determined unconsciously, the critical importance of early experience in this respect, and the underlying information dynamics that drive the whole thing – all of this is perfectly in line with Freud's account of the mental apparatus. There is almost no aspect of our current understanding of how the brain works, in big-picture terms, that is inconsistent with what he sketched out a century ago, by psychoanalytically 'dissecting the function'.

I don't want to imply that we have accomplished nothing at all in the years since. It's true that much of what we know today was rediscovered independently of Freud. Notwithstanding his early insights into the neuron, large parts of modern neuroscience – such as the vast field of molecular neurobiology – are beyond anything he could plausibly have imagined. But our sense of being comprehensively *over* him obviously doesn't check out. He covered an awful lot of ground. We have spent a very long time retracing his steps, and that process is far from being complete. Enough of his basic insights were so clearly on the right track that it may be time to give his therapeutic recommendations a second look, too.

CHAPTER FOUR
The Talking Cure

ANALYST: What would you rather not remember?
PATIENT: It's a feeling that lasts forever. You can mess with a monkey without consequences. I mean a little monkey; not a baboon with fangs . . . I don't know why I have to remember this.
ANALYST: You're feeling it now, but it comes from back then. There's no one really threatening you now, not here. No one here will harm you. But still, you feel as if I might.
PATIENT: Life is like that.
ANALYST: Your life was like that once.
PATIENT: As a kid, in the streets, I could feel the jungle. There were all sorts of animals. With fangs and claws and all. What can I do?
ANALYST: Back then, you couldn't defend yourself.
PATIENT: I don't know any other way to be.
ANALYST: You're learning another way, right now.
PATIENT: From my side, I want to close my ears and eyes. Some people might have felt differently; I couldn't . . . I didn't develop the skill of fighting back. And after my childhood, I still can't talk back. That's why I have trouble speaking. [Silence.] To be honest, I am still remembering my brother, the shouting. I remember it in my body.
ANALYST: Can you tell me what you're remembering?
PATIENT: In my lungs, it's hard to breathe. My heart is pounding . . . It's stuffy in here. It's hard to breathe, the atmosphere is suffocating.

ANALYST: To survive in those conditions, back then, you retreated to the shed. Was it stuffy in there?
PATIENT: [Nods.]
ANALYST: Things are different now. Your brother is gone. And the shed: it no longer protects you – it restricts you. It keeps you from living your life.

— *From the author's clinical files*

Psychoanalytic training begins with your own personal analysis. When mine started with Clifford Yorke, my colleagues in the neurosurgery department asked me what it was for. Is it to determine your suitability? Is it an initiation? Aren't you worried about them brainwashing you? I was embarrassed: they seemed to equate psychoanalysis with scientology. I have to admit, though, I had some doubts of my own.

One's personal analysis continues throughout the training, alongside theoretical seminars and the longitudinal observation of a baby in its family environment, one assigned per candidate. From the third year onwards, these are supplemented by clinical seminars and the supervised treatment of a first training case. If you make adequate progress with that case, in your fourth year you may begin another one. If that goes well, too, then no less than one year later, you may ask to graduate. These are the minimum requirements. Very few candidates (as psychoanalytic trainees are called) complete their training within the minimum period. It usually takes at least six years.

The expensive part of the training is the cost of your personal analysis. I was lucky: Clifford Yorke charged candidates reduced fees, so I paid £30 per session (in 1980s money, admittedly).

The theoretical seminars were held at the Institute of Psychoanalysis in New Cavendish Street, just off Harley Street. They happened at night, since most candidates had day-jobs – as psychiatrists, clinical psychologists, social workers or psychotherapists, but some of them were anthropologists, philosophers, historians, and, in one of the cohorts behind me, a classical composer. I was the only neuropsychologist.

Psychotherapy treatments are usually conducted once or twice per week, face to face. Psychoanalysis proper entails three to five sessions per week, with the patient lying on a couch and the analyst seated behind them, according to the template laid down by Freud. This format had its origins in the fact that the therapy he practised first was hypnotism, where the patient was placed in a trance. When Freud ditched that for free association, he retained the *mise en scène* because he found that it facilitated introspection, and spared both patient and analyst from having to look at one another.

Each analytic candidate received the files of three patients who had applied for low-cost treatment at the London Clinic of Psychoanalysis, from which we were to choose whichever one seemed the most promising. A line in one of the files that I received caught my eye: 'will form a compliant and dependent transference'. To me, this meant that the senior analyst who assessed this patient predicted that she would stay the course. If my patient dropped out, that could add years to my training. So, I decided this 'compliant and dependent' individual was the one for me. Let's call her Mabel D.

I met her for an initial consultation at the Clinic, and we agreed to begin the analysis after the summer break, five sessions per week. Simple enough. Yet, when she arrived at the appointed time for our first session, she refused to lie on the couch. She was willing to proceed with the analysis, she said, but only if she could sit facing me. I explained that most people find it easier to not have to face their analyst while they look inwards and report their private thoughts, which can sometimes be embarrassing. 'I would rather be able to see you,' she insisted. It seemed that lying down made her feel vulnerable in some way.

So, we began like that: face to face. I asked her to report her thoughts and feelings to me and try to be as frank as possible. She looked down at her hands. Then she said quietly that difficult things had transpired over the summer break: her ex-boyfriend had contacted her out of the blue, from Ireland, and she didn't know how she felt about that. He had told her things about himself which, if they were true, were very scary. 'He bullies me,' she added, softly. 'I fear that I will never be able to leave him.' Then she was silent.

'What things did he tell you?' I asked, after a minute or two.

She responded aggressively to this, saying that I was pushing her to reveal things that could put her in danger. Recalling what I had learnt about 'transference', I suggested that perhaps it felt like *I* was bullying her now. In response to this, she shouted, 'I don't want to play your fucking linking games!' So much for compliance.

Over the next few months, Mabel D subjected me to a barrage of suspicion, accusation and attack. During some sessions, she refused to say a word for the entire 50 minutes. Once she brought a newspaper along, read it silently to herself for the full analytic hour, and then left. On other days, she refused to leave the Clinic at the end of a session; then I would take her to the waiting room and stay in the entrance hall until she felt safe enough to go outside.

So it went on, month after month: moments of extreme vulnerability intermixed with endless unreasonable demands. I had never known anything like it. What it resembled, I learnt years later, was becoming a parent for the first time: the baby still there with its boundless needs, day after day. But this patient was evidently a very unwell baby.

What made her analysis especially taxing was that I found it almost impossible to empathize with her. She thought and behaved in such a perverse and self-defeating way that she was more maddening than pitiable. Almost everything she said and did was irrational to me. She was incomprehensible. Fortunately, my supervisor, Eglé Laufer, didn't have the same difficulty: my patient's illogic seemed to make sense to her. Still, I had only one supervision session per week, and the understanding that Laufer provided me with quickly fizzled out during the following session, which meant that I had to fly blind for four analytic sessions out of every five.

A further challenge was that my supervisor thought Mabel D was attracted to me. As a confident young man in my twenties, this didn't immediately strike me as absurd, but Laufer's theory had some convolutions that gave me pause. She claimed that my patient experienced her attraction to me as frightening, and therefore experienced me as frightening and sexually threatening. This is called 'projection'. The theory might sound plausible when you read about it in a book; but I was now being asked to seriously suggest to the frightened young woman sitting in front of me that the real reason she felt threatened was because she desired me physically. This seemed implausible, not to mention misogynistic, so I implemented Laufer's recommendations with very little confidence. I shouldn't have doubted her: the patient's response to my tentative suggestion that she might have sexual feelings toward me quickly convinced me that my supervisor was right.

Within a year, Mabel D declared that she was ready to begin using the couch. Just two sessions later, she confessed that she feared I might be masturbating behind her. It was very difficult for her to persevere through this anxiety; but she did, and she continued to freely associate, returning by and by to childhood memories. She recalled her father coming home from work, when he would read the newspaper in the sitting room. She was never sure what he was doing behind that newspaper. At the very least, she said at last, he might have had an erection. This thought led to several disturbing memories of other childhood thoughts she had had about him. I began to wonder whether Mabel's father had abused her sexually.

Then, one day, she told me something that she had never told anyone before. When she was very young – she couldn't work out how young – she had been fondled genitally by an uncle (her father's brother), who was babysitting her. She knew that what he did was wrong, but she never told her parents about it. She was afraid of their anger, especially her mother's. This fondling by the uncle happened repeatedly, sometimes accompanied by him masturbating himself. It ended only when Mabel's father died, when she was 12 years old, after which her mother re-married and they moved from a small rural village to the city of Dublin.

It took months for Mabel to tell me the worst of it. She 'confessed' that she was not only disgusted and frightened but also *stimulated and excited* by what happened at the hands of her uncle. He had said that it was their secret, and it was. Then she blurted out: 'maybe I brought it upon myself from the start'.

When I reassured her that it was nonsensical to believe that she – as a toddler – had somehow seduced her uncle, Eglé Laufer told me I had made a technical mistake. It was important, she explained, for the patient to know that I understood the ambiguity of her feelings, otherwise I couldn't help her with the shame and guilt. So, the next time Mabel expressed doubt about whether she was partly to blame, I said that my reassuring her on that score might make her feel alone with her doubts; and she agreed. Still today, she said, she imagined herself telling her mother (by then a 60-year-old widow), and her mother slaps her across the face for doing such disgusting things.

This led Mabel to confess something else to me. Sometimes, she said – even though she knows it is crazy to think like this – she finds herself wondering whether *any* of it really happened.

Isn't all of this just creepy nonsense? Haven't I described some weird ritual after all? Did that mumbo-jumbo about 'projection' really cure anybody? How is the process that I have just described different from other occult scams? What did I actually do that made Mabel better, and how do I know that it did? Didn't I just sit there while she sorted herself out? And *did* she sort herself out? Don't they say that you never are really cured by talking therapy? And didn't Mabel herself say that she wasn't sure whether what she remembered really happened? Anyway, the part where I told her that it was her own fault for being afraid of me – that she was afraid of me because she was sexually attracted to me – that seemed downright abusive. Isn't that what Freud did: bully his patients into accepting perverted interpretations of their distress?

These are serious questions. My answer to them comes down to three things: (1) We now have very good evidence that this stuff works. (2) We have – and we have had for a century – an explanation in Freudian terms for why. (3) We now have good evidence that those Freudian terms were basically right, given what we have discovered about the brain and how it changes itself.

As we saw, when Saul Rosenzweig wrote to Freud to report 'experimental verification' of his repression theory, Freud's unfortunate response convinced his followers that psychoanalysis was above such things. Freud said that 'the wealth of reliable observations on which these assertions rest make them independent of experimental verification'. Then he went on to say: 'Still, it [experimental verification] can do no harm'.[1]

Unfortunately, many of his followers seemed to feel that it *would* be a mistake to test their techniques experimentally, because the effects are too complex, too subjective, too profound, or too subtle to be reduced to mere numbers. The psychoanalyst Carlo Strenger, for example, contended recently that 'psychoanalysis properly belongs outside the realm of natural science and, hence, should not be judged by the same criteria'. He argues that psychoanalytic theory and practice are not concerned with scientific facts and figures, but rather with 'interpreting the structure of meaning'. Thus, psychoanalytic treatment yields 'a collection of persuasive story lines that assist analyst and patient to find meaning in the patient's symptom'.[2] You cannot *measure* such things, the argument goes.

Meanwhile, the proponents of many other forms of therapy (almost all of them derived from psychoanalysis) leapt at the chance of scientific validation. The best-known example is 'cognitive behavioural therapy' (CBT).* Having obtained scientific validation, they could say their approaches were 'evidence based',

---

*   Aaron Beck, the founder of CBT, was a psychoanalyst originally. He trained at the Philadelphia Psychoanalytic Institute between 1954 and 1960, but when he graduated, his application for membership of the American Psychoanalytic Association was rejected (twice) – due to the evaluating committee's scepticism about his claims of success from relatively brief treatments. He was advised to undertake additional supervised clinical work, which delved more deeply into the origins of his patients' symptoms, but he refused to do so.

in contrast with psychoanalysis, which was not. As a result, by the time the psychoanalysts of my generation finally got around to testing the original method properly, the horse had bolted.

This had three consequences. First, the established standards for measuring treatment outcomes were defined mainly in cognitive and behavioural terms. I'll have more to say later about how mental disorders might better be characterized; for now, let's just say that I wouldn't start with cognition and behaviour, but this is where we are, because analysts in their purity decided to sit out the crucial discussions. Second, the dosages and durations (i.e., the number and frequency of sessions) used in cognitive-behavioural treatments became the standard against which competing therapies are compared. So, in effect, the main point of comparison between treatments has become *cost efficiency*; not, say, long-term effectiveness, or whether they suppress the symptoms but leave the causes untouched, to say nothing of whether the storylines that supposedly assisted the patients to find 'meaning' were persuasive or not. Third – most trivial but in some ways most pernicious – the phrase 'evidence based' became linked, seemingly permanently, to the approaches that welcomed experimental scrutiny first (i.e., psychopharmacology and CBT), even though the psychoanalytic approach turned out later to be equally evidence based.[3] Therefore, when healthcare funders today say that they support 'evidence based' treatments for psychiatric disorders, what they typically mean is that they *do not* support psychoanalysis.

In a widely cited article, upon which much of what I will say in this chapter is based, my colleague Jonathan Shedler put it like this:

> There is a belief in some quarters that psychodynamic concepts and treatments lack empirical support or that scientific evidence shows that other forms of treatment are more effective. The belief appears to have taken on a life of its own. Academicians repeat it to one another, as do healthcare administrators, as do healthcare policymakers. With each repetition, its apparent credibility grows. At some point, there seems little need to

question or revisit it because 'everyone' knows it to be so. The scientific evidence [however] tells a different story.[4]

When testing medical treatments, the gold standard is what's called a *double-blind randomized controlled trial*.

'Controlled' means that patients receiving the treatment under investigation are compared with a 'control' group that is *not* receiving that treatment, so you can see whether the treatment is better than nothing. In drug research, the control group usually receives a placebo, but it can mean also that they receive no treatment at all, or that they remain on a waiting list initially but then receive the treatment later, or that they receive a competing treatment (in which case they are called a 'comparison' group), or that they receive the treatment they were receiving already (which is called 'treatment as usual').*

'Double-blind' means that neither doctor nor patient knows which treatment is being administered. The point of this is to avoid the placebo effect: very often, *believing* in a treatment can enhance its actual efficacy, and vice-versa. Obviously, it is easier to 'blind' doctors and patients in psychopharmacology than in psychotherapy research: just use two identical-looking pills, one of which is the real drug and the other a placebo, without the doctor or the patient knowing which is which. In practice, it isn't quite so simple: doctors and patients frequently know which pill is which, for instance because only one of them shows the expected

---

* All therapies – including physical ones like bone-setting techniques, or whatever – require a bit of thought to test against a control technique. Do you leave the control group's broken bones untreated, for example? But creating a control condition to compare with a talking therapy poses special challenges. How do you design a talking therapy that definitely doesn't do anything? Must the control group and their therapists not talk? How do you ensure that the therapists who provide a sham treatment don't know they are delivering a placebo? And what would motivate patients to stick with such treatments, which, prima facie, aren't helpful?

side effects. For this reason, researchers sometimes use 'active' placebos (that is, drugs that do *something*, but not the thing that the treatment does). In other cases, two competing pharmaceuticals or psychotherapies may be compared directly with each other. Still, there is no obvious way to be 'blind' as to what form of psychotherapy you are receiving, let alone administering.

'Randomized' means that patients are randomly allocated to either of the two treatments. This is meant to ensure that, aside from which of the treatments they actually receive, there are no important aggregate differences between the two groups. (If one group chooses psychoanalysis because they believe in psychoanalysis, for example, that might well distort the outcome of the trial.)

People who participate in randomized trials must be informed that they might receive a sham treatment, which further reduces the placebo effect. However, it is easier to persuade patients to participate in a drug trial lasting just a few weeks (when they know they might receive a placebo, and, if they do, they will receive the real treatment later) than it is to persuade them to participate in a psychotherapy trial which typically lasts several months – and really *should* last several years, but doesn't. When two different approaches to psychotherapy are compared with each other, patients frequently object to being randomized, since they have a preference for one of the two treatments – which is precisely why they must be randomized in the first place.

These problems were all solved, one way or another, by researchers of 'evidence based' psychotherapies – at least to the satisfaction of the healthcare providers and funders. By the time that researchers of psychoanalysis joined the race, they simply had to follow the established protocols and practices. In the single biggest comparative study between psychoanalysis and CBT, for example, patients in each treatment group who refused to be randomized were compared not only with each other but also with those who were willing to be randomized, and the data was processed by an independent team of 'blind' statisticians that was appointed by the analysts and the CBT practitioners, jointly, in advance.[5] We may therefore trust that apples were properly compared with pears when we look at the results of these studies in the aggregate, and observe the surprisingly strong patterns that have emerged.

First, though, a final piece of statistical jargon. 'Effect size' is a measure of the *magnitude* of a therapeutic effect. It tells you how powerful a treatment is, in a way that allows different treatments (and, very importantly, different experiments) to be compared with one another. That common metric is called a 'standard deviation'. On a graph, a bell curve represents a normally distributed population, so bell curves apply pretty much everywhere that you might intuitively imagine there to be a 'normal' way to be. For any suitable characteristic you can measure (height, for instance), the *average* person is situated in the middle of the curve. This middle point is called the 'mean', which is the highest point on the curve because that is where the largest number of people are located. The mean of a normal population is also called the '50th percentile', because it indicates that the average person has a score that is better than 49.9% of the population and worse than the other 49.9%.

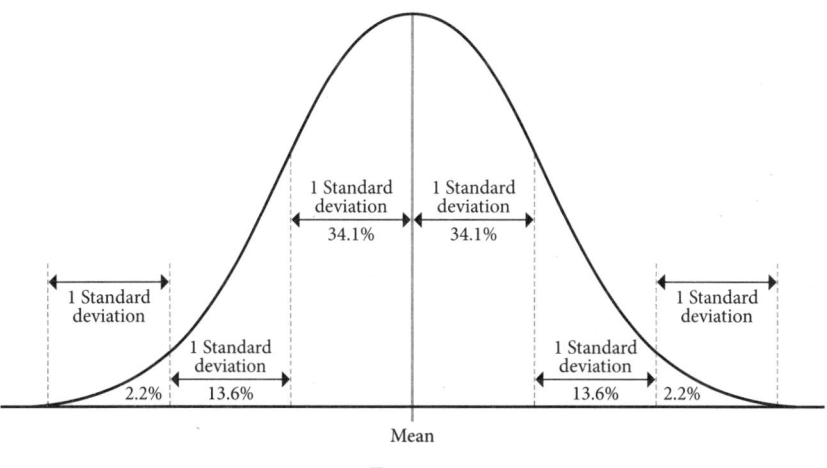

Figure 1

Now, suppose that the curve plots the distribution of some measure of suffering among people with depression (usually, the Beck Depression Inventory). The further left you look, the worse a time the test subjects are having. The further right you look, the better. People in the middle of the chart are suffering from their depression by the average amount.

If a medication shifts the average score of the treatment group to a position one standard deviation higher than that of the control group, this indicates that, on average, people who received the medication now feel better than 84.1% of those who did not (since 50% + 34.1% = 84.1%; see Figure 1). We call this shift from the 50th to the 84th percentile an 'effect size' of 1, because the size of the shift is one *standard deviation*. If a drug shifts the score two standard deviations above the control group's mean, it indicates that, on average, people who received the treatment feel better than 97.7% of those who did not (since 84.1% + 13.6% = 97.7%; see Figure 1). This is an effect size of 2. And if the shift is to make the average score better than 99.9% of the control group's mean (97.7% + 2.2% = 99.9%), this is an effect size of 3.

By convention, any medical treatment with an effect size of 0.80 (i.e., almost 1 standard deviation) is considered *highly* effective. Any treatment with an effect size of 0.50 is considered *moderately* effective. Any treatment with an effect size of 0.20 is considered *slightly* effective.[6] An effect size of 0.00 means, of course, that there is no difference between the treatment and control groups: the treatment is not effective at all.

Let's look at some comparisons. Viagra (a treatment for erectile dysfunction) has an effect size of 0.38; so, it is considered moderately effective. Antihypertensive drugs (for high blood pressure) have effect sizes of between 0.54 and 0.58: so, moderately effective. Corticosteroids for asthma have effect sizes of between 0.45 and 0.66: moderately effective. Sleeping pills (benzodiazepines and zolpidem for chronic insomnia) have an effect size of 0.30: slightly effective. Ibuprofen (for pain) has an effect size of 0.14; nicotine patches (against smoking) have an effect size of 0.18; and statins (for high cholesterol) have effect sizes of between 0.13 and 0.17. All these latter medications are only slightly effective, but we probably wouldn't want to be without them. When used as a heart attack preventative, aspirin has an effect size of just 0.02. Still, it's considered worth taking in most cases.*

Now, let's consider psychotherapy.

For research purposes, 'psychotherapy' is typically defined as talking therapy – two people just talking to each other – in other words, we are considering one or another of the many treatments that ultimately derive from psychoanalysis. In these terms, how effective is it? There are of course many different types of psychotherapy, and they yield different outcomes with different mental disorders. It would take another book to discuss every psychopathology in relation to every type of therapy; but here are the big-picture results, from the most widely cited and reputable sources.

The first major review of psychotherapy's overall effectiveness took place in 1980.[7] A meta-analysis is a principled way of drawing broader conclusions from overlapping pieces of statistical research: if you want to know how good a heart medication is, you naturally want to know what *all* the relevant studies found, not just one of them, and you want your survey to take some account of the differences between the studies, logically and transparently weighting them according to their methods, sample sizes and so on. The 1980 review was a meta-analysis of this kind: it included 475 studies, with a wide range of diagnoses, covering various approaches to psychotherapy. It found an overall effect size of 0.85.

A subsequent meta-analysis looked specifically at outcomes in the treatment of depression,[8] and summarized the findings of 37 psychotherapy studies. It found an overall effect size of 0.73. A very influential review published three years later[9] tabulated the results

---

* The definition of 'effect size' that I've just provided is called the 'between subjects' effect, because it compares two different groups of people: those who did and those who did not receive a treatment. In this chapter, unless I say otherwise, this is the kind of effect size I am talking about. However, some studies use a different definition of effect size. This is called the 'within subjects' effect, because it compares a group of people with itself: before and after the treatment. This second kind is less precise, since it is difficult to determine whether the measured effect was due to the treatment alone. (There might have been other variables that caused the change, such as spontaneous remission.)

of 18 *meta-analyses* of psychotherapy outcome studies. It yielded an average effect size of 0.75. So, overall, the generally recognized figure for psychotherapy outcome studies is that they show effect sizes of between 0.73 and 0.85. Highly effective. As a treatment, its effectiveness is comparable to that of oral hypoglycaemics for type 2 diabetes.

Drug therapy and psychotherapy trials can't be compared precisely, for all the methodological reasons we have discussed. Yet the gap in effectiveness that has emerged isn't of a scale so small that improvements in precision are likely to change the picture very much. SSRIs, the most widely used antidepressant medications, have an average effect size of 0.31: less than half as effective against depression as psychotherapy.[10] The same applies to ECT, which has an effect size of 0.29.[11] The most widely used anti-anxiety medications (benzodiazepines) have an average effect size of 0.38.[12] The average effect size for antipsychotic medications (for the treatment of schizophrenia) is 0.47.[13] (The average effect size for adjunctive treatment of schizophrenia by psychotherapy is 0.40.)[14] In other words, whereas psychotherapy in general is 'highly effective', the most common psychiatric medications are only 'moderately effective'. (A notable exception is methylphenidate, which is widely used for the treatment of ADHD. The average effect size for this medication is 0.90. On the other hand, it's a somewhat risky drug that can have unpleasant side effects, and it works only while you're taking it. Then again, the same could be said about antipsychotics, which are only half as effective.)

Enough about psychotherapy in general. Let's get back to the original brand. What about good old-fashioned psychoanalysis?

The most rigorous meta-analysis was published in 2006 in the Cochrane Library, a highly regarded independent authority on the efficacy of medical treatments of all kinds.[15] Its review included 23 randomized controlled trials of short-term psychoanalytic[16] therapy (where 'short-term' meant approximately 40 sessions), in 1,431 patients, with a wide range of common psychiatric disorders. Most psychoanalysts consider 40 sessions to be too few to make a real difference: it's less than two months of treatment at the standard pace, and one year at a rate of one session per week. Nevertheless, this survey yielded an overall effect size of 0.97 for general symptom improvement. And when patients were examined again after the end of their treatment (nine months later, on average) the effect size *went up* to 1.51. That's puzzling, isn't it?

In case you're wondering whether the Cochrane meta-analysis properly accounted for 'regression to the mean', otherwise known as 'people just getting better naturally over time', it did: this huge effect size shows how much better the treated patients were than those who were left to get better by themselves.*

What I have described is the single most highly regarded meta-analysis, but it is by no means the only one.†

---

* The meta-analysis also looked at change in three specific categories of symptom. This part of the study yielded an effect size of 0.81 for improvement in somatic symptoms, which increased to 2.21 at follow-up; an effect size of 1.08 for improvement in anxiety symptoms, which increased to 1.35 at follow-up; and an effect size of 0.59 for improvement in depressive symptoms, which increased to 0.98 at follow-up.

† In 2014 the Cochrane meta-analysis was updated to include 10 more randomized control trials of short-term psychoanalytic psychotherapy (Abbass et al., 2014). It now found an overall effect size of 0.71, and, again, this *increased* to 1.51 at long-term follow-up. A second highly regarded meta-analysis, published in the *Archives of General Psychiatry*, included 17 high-quality randomized controlled trials of short-term psychoanalytic therapy (Leichsenring, Rabung & Leibing, 2004). The average dosage was even lower than in the Cochrane Library meta-analysis (just 21 sessions). Nevertheless, this study yielded an effect size of 1.39, which increased to 1.57 at long-term follow-up (13 months post-termination, on average). These are extremely impressive numbers. Translating the effect size into percentage terms, the authors noted that patients treated with short-term psychoanalytic therapy were 'better off with regard to their target problems than 92% of the patients before therapy'. A third highly regarded meta-analysis, reported in the *American Journal of Psychiatry*, examined the efficacy of both psychoanalytic psychotherapy (14 studies) and CBT (11 studies) for personality disorders (Leichsenring & Leibing, 2003). The meta-analysis reported effect sizes using the longest follow-up periods available in the published scientific literature. For short-term psychoanalytic therapy (where the typical length of treatment was 37 weeks), the average follow-up period was 1.5 years. The effect size for psychoanalytic psychotherapy was again found to be extremely high, namely 1.46. For CBT (where short-term treatment

What about *long-term* psychoanalysis? In the real world, psychoanalytic treatments are typically conducted for more than one year. A meta-analysis reported in the *Journal of the American Medical Association*[17] compared long-term psychoanalytic psychotherapy (defined as 50 sessions, on average) with short-term therapies, for the treatment of multiple or chronic mental disorders or personality disorders. This study yielded an effect size for long-term psychoanalytic psychotherapy of 1.80 for overall outcome. Again, the effect size increased at long-term follow-up (an average of 23 months post-treatment). A second meta-analysis, reported in the *Harvard Review of Psychiatry*,[18] examined the effectiveness of long-term psychoanalytic therapy (defined as 150 sessions, on average) for adult outpatients with a range of diagnoses. For patients with mixed/moderate pathology, the effect size was 0.78 for general symptom improvement. This increased to 0.94 at long-term follow-up (an average of 3.2 years post-treatment). For patients with severe personality pathology, the effect size was 0.94. This increased to 1.02 at long-term follow-up (an average of 5.2 years post-treatment). A subsequent study of long-term psychoanalytic therapy for the treatment of chronic depression, which is still in progress (but interim results for which were published in the *Canadian Journal of Psychiatry* concerning outcomes three years after the commencement of the treatment)[19] shows even better results. The reported effect sizes, which increased with each additional year of treatment, were between 1.62 and 1.89, after three years of therapy. Again, these are off-the-charts numbers. (However, the last study used a 'within subjects' definition of effect size, and follow-up data are not yet available from this ongoing study.)

Against this background, a systematic review In *Lancet Psychiatry*[20] of 64 randomized controlled trials of both short-term *and* long-term psychoanalytic psychotherapy focused on the question

---

is considered normal, and the typical length of treatment was 16 weeks), the average follow-up period was 13 weeks. (Shorter follow-up periods, like shorter treatments, is normal for CBT.) The effect size for CBT was again found to be impressive – namely 1.00 – but not as impressive as for psychoanalytic therapy.

of 'equivalence'. Could psychoanalytic treatments be considered at least as effective as (or no less effective than) other evidence-based treatments, such as CBT and psychopharmacology? The review concluded that psychoanalytic psychotherapy is equivalent to all other treatments with established efficacy in respect of all the psychiatric disorders that were studied, with the single exception of cocaine dependence, for which drug counselling is better. (It *would* be cocaine: Freud's notorious weakness.)*

If psychoanalytic therapy weren't *at least* as effective as CBT, it would be difficult to understand the finding that when CBT practitioners need therapy for themselves, they mostly choose psychoanalytic therapy.[21]

Here is the bottom line. According to the standard medical definition, even relatively brief psychoanalytic treatments may be safely described as 'highly effective', and not by a narrow margin: taking follow-up scores into account, for certain conditions, even short courses of psychoanalysis seem as dependable as, say, insulin is at managing type 1 diabetes, or the HPV vaccine is at preventing cervical cancer. Most strikingly, there is a consistent finding that the improvement in symptoms endures at follow-up, and also that patients who receive psychoanalytic psychotherapy *continue to improve* after the termination of the therapy.

This is called the 'sleeper effect', and it is very interesting indeed. It seems to occur only with psychoanalytic therapy; even relatively similar psychotherapies don't show it to anything like the same degree. The natural inference is that the *causal* mechanism of psychoanalytic therapy must somehow keep going after the treatment has ended, so that the patient continues to accrue benefits. But what mechanism could that be?

On this question, we find that Freudian theory and modern neuropsychology are so closely aligned that you could hardly get a cigar leaf between them.

---

* The joke is wearing thin. The fact is, there is no convincing evidence that Freud ever was dependent on cocaine. He used it in small doses only, and for a brief period, about ten years before he developed his psychoanalytic theories (see Lebzeltern, 1983).

When Freud wrote to Fliess in 1896 that what was essentially new about his theory was 'the thesis that memory is present not once but several times over, that it is laid down in various kinds of indications', he included this drawing with his letter:[22]

```
                I        II       III
   W           Wz        Ub       Vb        Bews
 x  x———x  x———x  x———x  x———x  x
    x      x  x       x        x         x
                      x
```

Figure 2

'*W*' stands for perception, '*Wz*' stands for perceptual trace, and then came Freud's three main memory systems: '*Ub*' (unconscious); '*Vb*' (preconscious) and '*Bw*' (conscious). In the standard model of memory that is used in neuropsychology today, these three systems have been given different names, but they still stand in the same functional relation to each other:

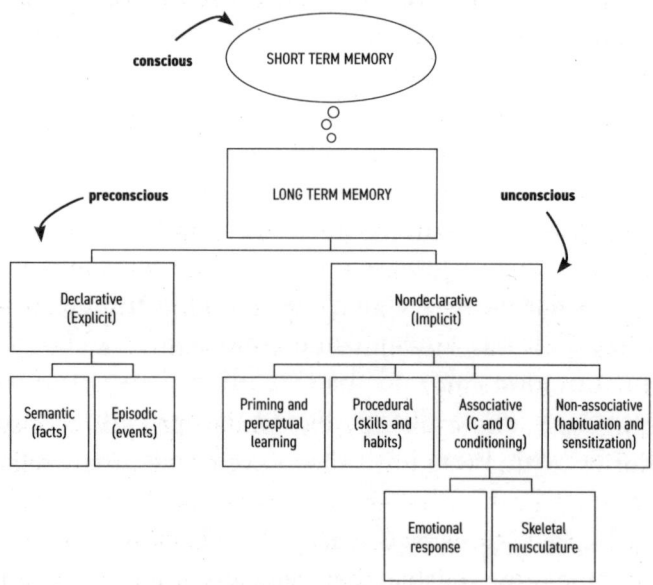

Figure 3

The first system is called 'short-term memory'. Freud called it 'consciousness'; and consciousness is its defining feature. The information held in this system is what you are aware of *right now*. Its capacity is remarkably limited: on average, our mind's eye can cope with only seven chunks of information at any given moment. For this reason, the long-term memory systems have to do most of the heavy lifting in day-to-day existence.

So, your short-term memory is constantly decanting its contents into the second major system – in a process called 'consolidation'. This second system is called 'declarative' long-term memory, since its contents can be, well, declared. Because information held in it can be brought back to consciousness (that is, back into short-term memory), Freud called it the 'preconscious' system.

Why do we sometimes need to return memories to conscious awareness? The point of memory is to tell us what the world is like. Memories guide us through recurring places and situations. They record what seem like the structural features of reality, and also where we last saw our keys. They are, in effect, predictions. Memories are *about* the past but they are *for* the future. It is only when 'prediction error' occurs that we need to bring the faulty memory back to consciousness, to be revised in light of the event that caught us out. Once we have fixed it, it can be 'reconsolidated' back into declarative long-term memory.

Freud said that 'consciousness arises *instead of* a memory trace'. Physiologically, as we now know, the process of reconsolidation literally dissolves long-term memory traces and returns them to a state of lability.[23] Your midbrain squirts neuromodulator chemicals up into the cortex, where the synaptic connections storing the memory trace that has suddenly lit up physically dissolve, because it turned out to be wrong.

Learning works by cyclically consolidating and reconsolidating memories in this way until they have proven their reliability. When we don't know what we are doing, we keep revising our preconscious predictions by bringing them back to consciousness. As they become more reliable, they need less attention. That means they spend more time in the second memory system, operating automatically and non-consciously. A lesson that you've learned is one you don't have to think about, and you think about it less and less the better you've learned it.

The third and last major memory system is called 'nondeclarative' because its contents cannot be declared, which means they cannot be brought back into consciousness.* This is what Freud famously called 'the unconscious'. In popular culture there seems to be an idea that – if it exists at all – it is an Oz-like shadow realm full of trippy detritus, memories grown weird and monstrous through avoidance. For the most part, it is the exact opposite. The contents of the nondeclarative memory system are predictions assumed to be so reliable, and so constantly in service, that it makes sense to save them in the brain's most efficient read-only format. But the 'read-only' analogy is misleading in one important respect: unlike declarative memories, these memories are not *images* which can be brought to mind and held there while we think about them; rather, they are *policies* – behavioural responses – that are 'remembered' only through being *enacted*. Unconscious memories are experiences that have become infrastructure, automatic as reflexes.

Here is a typical statement of how modern neuropsychologists tend to view matters:

> To consciously and wilfully regulate one's own behaviour, evaluations, decisions, and emotional states requires considerable effort and is relatively slow. Moreover, it appears to require a limited resource that is quickly used up, so conscious self-regulatory acts can only occur sparingly and for a short time. On the other hand, the non-conscious or automatic [psychological processes . . .] are unintended, effortless, very fast, and many of them can operate at any given time. Most important, they are effortless, continually in gear, guiding the individual safely through the day.[24]

---

* You will notice in Figure 3 that it is also called 'implicit' memory. The distinction between 'explicit' and 'implicit' in modern neuropsychology is identical with Freud's distinction between 'manifest' and 'latent'.

Freud said basically the same thing, 100 years earlier.

I have said that declarative and nondeclarative memories are encoded in different formats. They are also stored in different brain structures. The former are housed in the cerebral cortex; the latter are entered into brain regions *under* the cortex (mainly the basal ganglia and cerebellum, but also the amygdala and other subcortical emotional circuitry).[25] These brain systems brook no delay. They function by means of what Freud called the 'primary process': their output is rapid, highly stereotyped, and cannot be checked against experience: the so-called 'secondary process' has been cut out of the loop. Unrestrained by incoming error signals, the action patterns of your nondeclarative memory systems are fixed, for life. You can always add new ones, but you can't get rid of the ones you already have.

Today, we divide declarative and nondeclarative long-term memory into further subsystems. The most superficial of these is 'episodic' declarative memory. Episodic memories take the form of movies in your head. We commonly use memories like these to guide ongoing decision-making in uncertain situations. For example, if I am trying to find a destination that I visited once before, I replay the movie to see how I got there last time.

The next most superficial subsystem is called 'semantic' declarative memory. Semantic memories also take the form of images, but they are less concrete than episodic ones: they take the form not so much of first-person experiences as third-person generalizations. If I visit the same destination several times, such as the hospital where I work, it is inefficient for me to play movies depicting every previous occasion I went there. Rather, I average those many episodes into one abstract schema: *Take the R45. Turn left onto the R310. When you reach Stellenbosch, take Baden Powell Drive,* and so on.

(The talking that goes on in the talking cure happens in words, of course, but the words are used initially to retrieve and describe experiences – memories, thoughts, feelings and the like – so, they are 'episodic' to begin with. It takes time for the deeper patterns to emerge – generalized insights about yourself that can be consolidated into 'semantic' memory.)

The third level of consolidation takes us into the nondeclarative subsystems. All of these processes operate simultaneously, but the spadework of day-to-day life gradually shifts from the declarative to the nondeclarative systems. When I drive to work these days, I don't need to hold the 'semantic' memory in my mind: I drive there *automatically*, using the nondeclarative subsystem that is called 'procedural' memory. This automatized function is a valuable efficiency because it frees my short-term memory to think about other things, like what to say to my boss when I walk through the door. But it has its drawbacks. Sometimes when I drive into Cape Town intending to go somewhere new, I find myself back at Groote Schuur Hospital, having gone there on autopilot.

Procedural memories are also called 'skills and habits' (see Figure 3). Who among us has no bad habits? All that is required for a behaviour to become habitual is for it to be performed many times. Whether they are good, bad, or indifferent, procedural predictions become automatized by brute repetition. In cognitive neuroscience we say that they are 'hard to learn and hard to forget'.

Yet bad habits can also be forged by a different mechanism.

Addiction evolved for good biological reasons, but it operates blindly. Attachment bonding, for example, which occurs during the first six months of life (and repeatedly thereafter, throughout life) is mediated by mu opioid receptors in the brain. The very same circuitry (in the 'emotional response' subsystem in Figure 3) can be triggered artificially using opiate drugs such as codeine, morphine or heroin. These substances are highly addictive, for the good biological reason that attachment bonding is absolutely essential. You *must* become addicted to your caregiver, and suffer withdrawal symptoms if they go AWOL. Yet if this brain circuitry is tricked, a person can become addicted to an artificial trigger in place of a *real* provider of love and care. The drug of abuse then 'stands in for' a real attachment figure. Doesn't all this sound rather Freudian? And yet, it is simply the current neuroscientific picture.[26]

This leads us to an important point about these memory systems: the nondeclarative ones are fully operational at birth, but the declarative ones are not. As a result, everything that you learned during the first two years of your life is totally unconscious and automatized and can never be reconsolidated in consciousness. The episodic and semantic memory systems come onstream only during the third year of life. This produces 'infantile amnesia'.

In the case of attachment bonding (for example), that's fine so long as you became attached to a good-enough caregiver in the first place. But some of us are not so lucky. What do you do if your only two choices are a violent father and a withdrawn mother? Naturally, you attach to the least bad option. But then, for the rest of your life, whenever you find yourself in need of loving care, your automatic response will be to look for somebody withdrawn. You have no idea that you are doing this, you have no control over it, and (for that very reason) you can't revise the original prediction that gave rise to it.

What's more, if this was your start in life, and the attachment figures you are attracted to aren't actually very good at caring for you, then the emotional need that draws you to them will go chronically unmet. This means that a *basic need* of yours goes unmet: a need that is found in all mammals, since all mammals need to be nursed. For this reason, a biological (homeostatic) alarm system goes off. Jaak Panksepp named this alarm system PANIC/GRIEF: it evolved to make us respond to separation and abandonment in a manner that maximizes our chances of survival.* It functions like the deepest kind of nondeclarative memory: a stereotyped action pattern, proven over aeons of evolutionary time. *First howl. Then give up.* (First 'protest', then 'despair', in the nomenclature of John Bowlby.[27]) Because this is an innate prediction – an instinct rather

---

* The capital letters, here and in other references to neurobiological drives, are Jaak Panksepp's own notation, indicating that we are talking about brain circuits *and* feelings.

than a memory – you don't know why you do it.* But the feeling pulls at you, all the time, somewhere beyond words.

A person with this start in life will have a high probability of suffering from major depressive disorder.²⁸ They will keep feeling the pain of separation and loss, and feel like throwing in the towel. And because nondeclarative memories can't be returned to consciousness, they will have no idea where their misery comes from.

Within the first few minutes of their initial consultation, patients seeking psychological help usually tell me what feeling it is they are struggling with. They might say something like: 'I don't know how to cope with social situations. I feel inept. I'm always on the outside; it's like everyone else knows what to do and say and I don't.'

Unwanted feelings are almost invariably what prompts people to consult psychotherapists in the first place. These feelings tell me *which of their emotional needs is not being met*. The aim of psychotherapy is always to help our patients find better ways of meeting their emotional needs. I am not embarrassed to put it so simply. The life of the mind is complicated, so it's a relief to be able to state some things plainly and simply.

When it comes to feelings (which are, never forget, conscious things), what you see is what you get. The psychoanalyst's initial task is not analysis, then, but classification. Freud called the property of being conscious 'our one beacon light in the darkness of depth psychology'.²⁹ So why not use it? The clinician's first job is to recognize the constellation of conscious complaints that the patient is *experiencing* and classify it accordingly.

The patient of mine whose presenting complaint was 'I don't

---

* The biological answer is: giving up (1) reduces the chances of alerting predators to the presence of an abandoned little one; (2) reduces the chances of the little one wandering too far from home base; (3) saves the little one's metabolic resources, which are in short supply in the absence of a caregiver.

know how to cope with social situations', was describing *social* anxiety. They went on: 'It's like everyone else knows what to do and say and I don't. This is also how it was when I was at school. I want to feel more confident. Even though I know that I've achieved a lot; still, I don't feel it. I want to be respected. To be honest: I want to be admired.' So, this patient was distressed about their social status. (Note the feeling words: confidence, achievement, respect, admiration.) Odd as it may sound, social status – no less than attachment bonding – is a basic mammalian need. Mammals are social animals; they live in groups, and their groups are organized hierarchically. The higher your rank in the pecking order, the greater access you have to the resources of the group. If you – mammal that you are – learn how to meet this need, you feel good in a particular way, and if you fail to meet it, you feel bad in a particular way – like this patient did.* The clinician's first job is to recognize the constellation of bad feelings – the *syndrome* – and to classify it accordingly.

In Freud's day, we had a very inadequate taxonomy of the basic needs of the human animal. Freud thought initially that all pleasures and unpleasures were *sexual*, so he ascribed their undeniable variety to what he called 'components' of a hypothetical, overarching sexual drive. The first such component drive was called 'oral' libido, the second was 'anal' libido, the third was 'phallic' libido and the fourth was 'genital' libido. Only the last of these is now recognized as sexual in the taxonomy of drives used in affective neuroscience.†

Freud would have classified the unmet need (the 'dispositional fixation', as he called it) of the patient we are discussing here as

---

* Think back to childhood. The playground was a jungle. Getting accepted into a 'cool' peer group and acquiring some status in the pecking order was a very important emotional task. Status matters no less to us adults; why else do we go to such lengths on social media, for example?

† There are still disagreements in contemporary neuroscience, of course, but our current taxonomies are at least based on identifiable brain circuits that can demonstrably be activated by specific brain chemicals.

that of phallic libido. (Mine is bigger than yours, and all that.) Those psychoanalysts who have kept up with developments in neurobiology, however – as Freud always expected us to do – would recognize this patient's emotional distress as an instance of frustrated PLAY (the mammalian need to feel accepted, included, confident, successful, respected, admired, etc.).

Once that is done, the puzzle becomes: why? Why does this patient suffer from this feeling in particular? There are always two sources of evidence. The first is the developmental history of the patient. Once I know which need is not being met, I listen to the patient's history with that in mind. How did they go about dealing with that need during their childhood? The answer can take some time to emerge, but at least I know what I am looking for. The second source of evidence is the patient's pattern of behaviour in their *current* emotional relationships. When someone keeps doing something that doesn't quite make sense, that's a big clue about how they grew up: just imagine the kind of context in which it *did* make sense.

Here's an example. A thirty-something woman with a diagnosis of borderline personality disorder came to me for help with relationship difficulties. She felt rejected and abandoned by her nearest and dearest, especially by lovers, but also by her closest friends. What soon became apparent was that she lurched from crisis to crisis, in a way that at first seemed unrelated to her relationship problems. Almost every week there was something new: she was involved in a motor vehicle accident, then she broke her arm by tripping on a paving stone, then she contracted COVID-19, then she dropped her mobile phone into a toilet, then she contracted COVID again, then she left her purse at a restaurant, and so on.

As her treatment continued, I gradually learned about her childhood. She was the second of three children. Her parents divorced when she was four years old, and she lived with her mother, a busy lawyer. Joining the dots in her memories, it became apparent that the only times that she got her mother's undivided attention was when she was in sufficiently serious trouble; when she fell ill, or failed an exam, or broke a toe. On this basis, I eventually inferred the repressed prediction: *the best way to obtain loving care is to have a crisis befall me.* This is typical of repressed predictions: they are silly and unrealistic, but they are also the best solution that the child could muster at the time. Once the prediction becomes automatized – that is, once the problem is 'put out of mind' – it is no longer subject to revision, even when the patient has grown up and could easily find better ways of obtaining loving attention. So, it becomes a recurring pattern of behaviour.

In our present example, this pattern was precisely the tendency to lurch from crisis to crisis; but it would not have been apparent to me that this pattern had anything to do with trying to obtain care and attention if I had not known that the feeling the patient suffered from was, essentially, separation distress.

Embedded within an emotional disorder is the patient's (unconscious) attempt to bring something about – specifically, to meet an emotional need. All symptoms of all disorders indicate underlying problems, but this is a further sense in which psychiatric symptoms *mean something*. When I first read Freud and trained as a psychoanalyst, I was told that psychiatric symptoms give expression to patients' repressed wishes. This never made sense to me. How could symptoms (which are unpleasant) express *wishes*? It was only later that I understood: what Freud called 'repressed wishes' are unrealistic childish predictions about how to meet an emotional need.

As it happens, this particular patient didn't remember thinking: 'The best way to gain my mother's attention is to get into trouble; so, from now on I am going to keep bringing disasters upon my own head'; that was an inference on my part. But inference is not always necessary: many patients make bad predictions of which they are perfectly aware, or of which they are capable of becoming conscious. These are what we call 'declarative' predictions, and what Freud called 'preconscious' wishes or 'phantasies'.* There are many things that we *can* think about but prefer not to. In such

---

* Psychoanalysts called fantasies 'phantasies', to differentiate them from conscious daydreams.

cases, the therapist's task is relatively simple: they must bring the faulty prediction to the patient's attention and *problematize* it. This gives the patient an opportunity to re-think it with the help of the therapist, and come up with a better solution.

Many forms of psychotherapy work like this, cognitive behavioural therapy (CBT) being only the best-known example. If the bad prediction is declarative, then the therapist's task is essentially to encourage the patient to take a deep breath and look at the facts in a new light. In CBT,[30] the therapist often goes further and suggests better predictions to the patient – even giving them 'homework' to practise putting these new solutions into effect. In many cases, this is all that is needed, which is why CBT achieves such good results.

But in other cases, the patient has no idea why they're doing what they're doing, or that it has anything to do with their suffering. What's more, they have no control over it, so they can't stop. This is because the prediction that generates the behaviour is *repressed*. 'Repressed', as Clifford Yorke informed me, doesn't mean 'I don't want to think about it'. It means 'I can't think about it'; the prediction is locked away in nondeclarative memory, where it must inexorably and involuntarily (and inexplicably) be repeated, not in ideas, but in actions.

This form of enactment is called *transference*. Many people (including many specialists) imagine that this term refers only to what patients think or feel about their therapists. In fact, transference to a therapist is no different from transference to a spouse or boss or friend or anyone else. Whenever we confront an emotional need that we couldn't master in childhood, we produce a stereotyped response (the 'least bad' one that we could come up with back then). This response is transferred from the past onto the present, as if the past were the same as the present.

The great value to the therapist of such enactments, however, is that they happen *now*. The repressed predictions can't be remembered from the past, but they can be *perceived* (when enacted) in the present, and therapists can draw their patients' attention to them, and make them aware of what they are doing.

In the old days, analysts thought it was necessary to be completely neutral and to behave indifferently toward their patients, so as not to 'contaminate' the transference: to create a blank screen upon which their patients could project their inner scripts. This explains a lot of what many people experienced as bizarre or scandalous conduct on the part of analysts. It used to be common practice, for example, for analysts to leave a gift given to them by a patient exactly where it was placed, session after session, until the patient gained enough 'insight' into their motivation to withdraw it. The critics were right: behaving like a robot isn't neutral; it's very odd. It is likely to provoke patients to respond in ways they typically would respond to cold and unsympathetic people, not necessarily how they typically responded to their parents or other significant others during childhood.

Anyway, you don't need to prompt transferences; on the contrary, you can't stop them. There is usually nothing very subtle about a pattern of behaviour that is automatically repeated right before your eyes. Mabel D, for example, couldn't suppress the suspicion that I was masturbating when I patently wasn't, and this both aroused and disgusted (and terrified) her, just as it did in childhood. Likewise, I unconsciously aped Clifford Yorke's limp, just as I had tried as a child to identify with my father, while resenting his making no effort to assist me in doing so. All you need do is draw the patient's attention to such things, and then link them with their symptoms. This is called 'transference interpretation', in which the therapist says something like this:

1. Can you see that you tend to respond to emotional situation X by doing Y, over and over again?
2. Can you see that this way of responding is meant to have outcome Z?
3. Can you see that it doesn't have that outcome?
4. Can you see that this is why you are suffering from the feeling that brought you to treatment?

When making point (2) it is helpful to use what you learnt from the developmental history of the patient, to put flesh on the bones of what is otherwise an abstract formula. So, for example: 'Can you see that losing your purse was meant to make your boyfriend pay more attention to you, *just like your mother paid more attention to you when you injured yourself as a child*?' Which leads to point (3): 'It didn't have the predicted result, did it? Instead, he became annoyed with you.'

When it's laid out schematically, as it is here, it's hard to imagine how such a conversation could be anything but irritating. And yet, in reality, patients don't seem to find it so. It is true that one's first attempt at an interpretation is often inaccurate, and the patient has to help you correct it. Once it clicks, though, it has an incredibly powerful effect. For the first time in their lives, their symptoms *make sense* to them. What is more, it becomes apparent to them that their suffering is – to some degree, at least – within their own hands. What they are *doing* is contributing to their distress. So, they must do something differently.

Case closed? Not yet, I'm afraid. Even when the patient fully accepts a transference interpretation, what invariably happens is that they still enact exactly the same behaviour again. So, you make the same interpretation again. Then, in the next session, you notice that the patient has done it again. And again, and again.

What else could one expect? The prediction is not erased just by drawing the patient's attention to its enactment. Because it is nondeclarative, it is stored in subcortical regions, in a format that cannot be altered by any amount of conscious effort. The patient therefore has no choice: they are not in control of these automatized systems. The best we can hope for is that they will gradually lay down a new and more realistic prediction *alongside* the old one.

For this reason, I frequently follow up the observation 'You did it again' by asking the patient how – on reflection – they might have dealt with the situation differently. The imaginative work of thinking it through helps them to lay down alternative predictions, a process that Freud pithily named 'working through'. In this respect, psychoanalytic therapists do not attempt to *teach* their patients new ways of meeting their needs. The aim of psychoanalytic therapy is to help our patients *find* new ways of meeting their emotional needs. We aim for nothing more than to free our patients from automaticity, from compulsion. (This is mainly because we don't know what the 'right' answer is for each and every person – which is ironic, considering that so many people experience us as know-it-alls.) But there is room for approaches like CBT that include prominent didactic components, too. Some people prefer to be shown the ropes by an expert, rather than to have to find their own way. And remember, CBT is all that's required in many cases; not every problematical prediction has its origins in earliest childhood.

That said, when the problem *is* a deeply unconscious one, it can be useful if the same interpretation is made in lots of different contexts. This helps the patient to see their pattern, but also to consolidate a different prediction that can be applied in a wide variety of situations. In this way, a number of different 'episodic' predictions gradually consolidate into a single 'semantic' one. And then, slowly but surely, the semantic one becomes more deeply consolidated, and it becomes a nondeclarative one: a new habit or a skill. Then the heavy lifting shifts to the unconscious systems, and the new prediction becomes as automatic as the old one was.

Why does the patient unconsciously shift from the old pattern to the new one? Simply because the new one *works*. It really does meet the underlying need, because it is the product of an adult mind, operating calmly and reflectively under very different circumstances from those that prevailed in childhood. Even so, the bad old ways are still there, in nondeclarative memory, and we can always go back to them, especially in times of stress. Unconscious predictions are indelible.

This also explains why psychoanalytic therapy takes *time*. Patients need many sessions at high frequency. It cannot be otherwise when it comes to nondeclarative memories, which are, after all, hard to learn and hard to forget. For patients who need kidney dialysis, it would be no good for a healthcare funder to restrict them to one session per month on grounds of affordability. That's not how the kidney works: the patients would get very ill and almost certainly die.³¹ It's the same for nondeclarative memory: this is simply how the subcortical brain works. Healthcare funders who want our treatments to produce quicker results are pushing against an immovable object. That's not how learning works.

How can you tell when the job is finished? Once the patient themselves reaches the point of recognizing that they are doing it again, *while they are doing it*, they don't need a therapist anymore. At that point, choice has replaced automaticity. This doesn't mean that the process of change comes to an end: 'working through' continues long after the end of the treatment. A patient who has gained insight into their repressed predictions gradually consolidates their new ones more deeply into nondeclarative memory, without needing the help of an analyst to do so. This explains the so-called 'sleeper' effect, in which patients who undergo psychoanalytic therapy continue to get *more better* after the end of their treatment. What was deliberate and artificial becomes unconscious and effortless: second nature.

This is what it means to be cured.

CHAPTER FIVE
Slips of the Tongue

> Two middle-aged women are taking tea together. They haven't seen each other for a while, and the conversation is somewhat stilted. Eventually, Mrs Brown plucks up the courage to confront Mrs Smith: 'I don't appreciate the fact that you told Mrs Jones my husband has a wart on the end of his penis.' 'I didn't tell Mrs Jones that your husband has a wart on his penis,' says Mrs Smith vehemently. 'I said it *feels* like he does.'
> — *Ancient proverb, source unknown*

When I began collecting material for my editorial job on the *Complete Neuroscientific Works of Sigmund Freud*, it became clear that I needed to read Freud's 1880s correspondence with his fiancée, Martha Bernays. In those years, he described his early research activities to her on an almost daily basis. To access these private letters, I needed the permission of Kurt Eissler. It was Eissler who set up the Sigmund Freud Archives at the Library of Congress in Washington, where he had recently resumed his directorship following the unhappy tenure of the (let's put it mildly) Freud sceptic, Jeffrey Masson.*

Given his experience with Masson, Eissler was wary enough to insist on an interview with me in person. The interview took place at his home in New York: a dark and cavernous apartment on Central Park West. He lived alone. His wife, Ruth, a fellow analyst

---

* For more on that story, and to get a sense of Eissler's personality, I highly recommend Janet Malcolm's book: *In the Freud Archives* (1984).

and a psychiatrist whom he had married in 1936, had died one year previously, and they had no children. He was almost 90 years old (born in 1908), tall and gaunt, and he had an unnerving way of looking through me – and sometimes over me – rather than at me. I learnt later that this was because he was almost blind, which presumably was also why his apartment was so dark; it made no difference to him.

The *New Yorker* journalist, Janet Malcolm, described him as a 'singular mixture of brilliance, profundity, originality, and moral beauty on the one hand, and wilfulness, stubbornness, impetuosity, and maddening guilelessness on the other'.[1] My own first impression of him was that he was frankly paranoid. He mistook my accent for Australian, and became suspicious when my responses to his rapid-fire questions made it clear that I knew none of the psychoanalytic people that one *should* know in Australia. Fortunately, his anxiety subsided when he realized that I was distantly related to the late Wilhelm Solms, a second-generation psychoanalyst who was president of the Vienna Psychoanalytical Society following the war, tasked with ensuring that Nazi collaborators were kept out.* Eissler told me with relish that my relative had said of the Austrians: 'They were terrible soldiers, but very good Nazis.'

Though I had never so much as spoken to this notable relation, it secured my approval with Eissler. From then on, I had the pleasure of being invited, every Friday evening when I was in New York, for a cognac-lubricated chat at his home. Eissler was the last surviving member of Freud's Vienna group, so this was the closest I ever came to meeting Freud himself.[2] We had extraordinarily edifying conversations, the memory of which I shall always cherish. He was a great connoisseur, not only of Freud, but also of Shakespeare and

---

* Wilhelm was above reproach; he was a well-known socialist whose nickname was *der rote Graf* ('the red Count'). Also, he shared the distinction with Eissler of caring for Freud's famous patient, the 'Wolf Man', during the latter's dotage in Vienna.

Goethe. It was Eissler who told me the joke about the old days, when even the future was better.

One of the things that struck me was how he spoke of psychoanalytic topics using Freud's original technical vocabulary, as if it was all literally true and nothing had changed since 1939. This stood in sharp contrast to what I was experiencing at the Institute of Psychoanalysis in London, which was essentially a Kleinian society by the time I trained there. This was another reason that Eissler didn't trust me initially; he assumed I was a disciple of Melanie Klein. He had a very low opinion of the Kleinians, and also, it seemed, of just about every school of psychoanalysis that deviated in any way from what Freud himself wrote – either in print or in his unpublished correspondences, which Eissler had preserved so assiduously for posterity.

When I remarked that the practice of psychoanalysis seemed to be changing in America, he took me to be saying that it was going to the dogs. So, he replied:

> I said the same thing to my analyst – Dr Aichhorn – after the horrors of the Second World War. He replied that he had said the same to Professor Freud after the First World War. So, you see Dr Solms, what you are telling me is what every generation of analysts says to the previous generation. The only difference is: this time you are right.

I only recall Eissler saying one critical thing about old-school psychoanalysis. He told me that he was suffering the 'incontinent nostalgia' of old age, which produced vivid childhood memories that were not previously available. It transpired that these memories contradicted some of Aichhorn's reconstructions of his early years. Eissler seemed genuinely shocked by this, a late suggestion of fallibility in the edifice to which he had dedicated his life.

No matter how out-of-time he seemed, I hung on his every word: trying to absorb as much as I could of that lost era, perhaps even to catch a trace (or at least an echo) of the personality of Freud himself. Eissler would always terminate our appointments after we had spoken for exactly 50 minutes, the mechanisms of procedural memory still ticking away with remarkable precision. Without glancing at his watch, the old man would get to his feet and gesture towards the door.

I don't remember the details of all my conversations with him. Yet, after one of them, in the winter of 1993, Eissler wrote to me:

Dear Doctor Solms,
   Thank you for the delightful hour. Analysis is in safe hands with you. [. . .]
   K. R. Eissler

His note supplied a good deal of much-needed courage when, two years later, I was appointed editor of the *Revised Standard Edition of the Complete Psychological Works of Sigmund Freud*.

This was a much more daunting task than just the neuroscientific papers, and the result, all 24 volumes of it, has taken me just short of three decades to complete.[3] Freud is already extremely controversial, and there is no 'correct' way to translate anyone, so I am sure to have made plenty of new enemies. (Jean Laplanche, for example, who oversaw the translation of Freud's complete psychological works into French, called my English predecessor's choice of the word 'anaclisis' for Freud's *Anlehnung* 'a lifeless and barbaric term'. Jim Underwood, a rival translator of Freud into English, accused my predecessor of 'throwing professional integrity to the winds' for using another neologism, 'cathexis'.)[4]

Even so, I don't regret taking on the mantle. There is no way to translate without asking yourself repeatedly, sentence by sentence, what the author is trying to say. What idea is entombed in these words? It creates a strangely intimate relationship – some days filial, some days parental, awe and exasperation chasing one another around the study.

Kurt Eissler died in 1999. In his cadences I could often hear Freud's voice. Later, poring over these century-old writings, the sound of it – solemnity tinged with irony – occasionally suggested a shade of meaning that might elude the everyday reader, even in the original German.

My point is, there might be nobody alive who has spent more time with Freud than I have.

Most of the controversies surrounding Freud's previous authorized translator, James Strachey, can be summarized in a single complaint: that he 'falsely scientized' his source.[5] The psychoanalyst Bruno Bettelheim argued that Freud's term *Seele* should have been translated 'soul' (rather than 'mind'), and that the title of his book *Die Traumdeutung* ('The Interpretation of Dreams') actually suggested 'divination' rather than interpretation. He argued that Freud, who allegedly had no truck with the strictures of polite society, would never have countenanced Strachey's rendering of *Kultur* as 'civilization'. But what most irked Bettelheim and his numerous allies was the way that Strachey translated everyday German words like *Besetzung*, *Ich*, *Es* and *Überich* using neologisms derived from ancient Greek and Latin: 'cathexis', 'ego', 'id' and 'superego' (in place of the colloquial 'occupation', 'I', 'it' and 'over me', respectively).[6]

I fear that this objection may reveal a lack of familiarity with the conventions of scientific writing in German and English. In German, it is normal to use everyday descriptive terms for things that in English science we denote by ancient Greek and Latin neologisms. What German chemists call *Wasserstoff* ('water stuff') and *Sauerstoff* ('sour stuff'), for example, we call 'hydrogen' and 'oxygen' in English. In neuroanatomy, Freud's primary discipline, German-speaking scientists denote a beam-like body of fibres that we call the 'corpus callosum' *das Balken* (the 'beam'), a bridge of fibres that we call the 'pons' *die Brücke* (the 'bridge'), and four bumps at the back of the midbrain that we call the 'corpora quadrigemina' *die Vierhügel* (the 'four hills'). A smallish part of the brain hanging off the back of the pons which we call the 'cerebellum', they have dubbed *das Kleinhirn* (the 'little brain'), to contrast it with what we call the 'cerebrum' (which they call *das Großhirn*, the 'big brain').

In this context, translating Freud's term *das Ich* (in its technical sense) as 'the I' would be a bit like translating *Sauerstoff* as 'sour stuff'. It might be interesting, but it would also be ridiculous, and it would sound less like science than it did when Freud wrote it. More to the point, it would sound less scientific than Freud intended it to be; and psychoanalysis has enough trouble on that score. I have already quoted Freud's remark to the effect that 'the deficiencies in our description [of the mental apparatus] would probably vanish if we were already in a position to replace the psychological terms by physiological and chemical ones'. He continued: 'It is true that they too are only part of a figurative language; but it is one with which we have long been familiar and which is perhaps a simpler one as well.'[7]

As is conventional in German science, Freud's technical vocabulary was for the most part everyday German deployed in a slightly unusual or extended way. Strachey's jargon is undeniably a piece of artifice, an intervention that may seem as radical and peculiar in its own way as one of Freud's dream analyses. For someone who feels, as I do, that Freud has been badly misunderstood, it sets a tempting example. While questions of basic terminology remain unresolved, would I not be justified in translating Freud's scientific German into an English that speaks to my scientific colleagues? The Freud whom I have come to know is, above all, a truth-loving scientist.

He is also a wordsmith. He writes with unusual clarity, without flourish, and he always bears in mind his reader's potential doubts and confusions, and then addresses them directly as he proceeds with his argument. From 1900 onwards, he never tires of explaining some points, no matter how many times he has done so before. This applies above all to his admirably patient explanations and justifications of his conclusion that 'mental' is not synonymous with 'conscious'. Indeed, it is precisely on this point that I sometimes find him annoying. He tells us again and again, like a patient enacting a transference, that the mental is unconscious 'in itself' (*an sich*). What does that mean? I can enlighten you, but only because he eventually explained it himself, in 1938, in a posthumously published essay titled 'An Outline of Psychoanalysis': Freud meant that the mind represents itself in the same way that it represents *external* things-in-themselves (in Kant's sense), namely, through the interface of phenomenal consciousness. To put it another way, your experience of your own mind is no more identical with the reality of your mind than your experience of a chair is identical with the chair's constituent atoms.

On other points, I cannot tell you what he means, because I would be guessing. Here is an example. Freud always insisted that, unlike ideas, feelings (also referred to as affects or emotions) are conscious by definition. Fair enough; but why? He explains:

> The whole difference arises from the fact that ideas are cathexes – basically of memory traces – while affects and emotions correspond to processes of discharge, the final manifestation of which are perceived as feelings.[8]

No? Me neither.

What is clear to me is that the overall trajectory of Freud's writing was a principled attempt to describe in *functional* terms what the brain looks like, or rather, how it works, when you study it from the subjective perspective.

In this book, I've already been using some Freudian terminology in quite free variation. *Functionalism* for 'metapsychology', *prediction* for 'wish', *prediction-error* for 'reality testing', *attachment figure* for 'love object', *automatized* for 'primary process', *declarative* for 'preconscious', *activation* for 'cathexis', and so on. Simply by doing a find-and-replace job on Strachey's translations, you can make Freud sound quite a lot like a 21st-century neuroscientist.

Here is an example, which might sound familiar to you:

> As a result of the link that has thus been established, next time this need arises a psychical impulse will at once emerge which will seek to re-cathect the mnemic image of the perception and to re-evoke the perception itself, that is to say, to re-establish the situation of the original satisfaction. An impulse of this kind is what we call a wish; the re-appearance of the perception is the fulfilment of the wish; and the shortest path to the fulfilment of a wish is a path leading direct from the excitation produced by the need to a complete cathexis of the perception.[9]

Here it is again, reconsolidated:

> As a result of the link that has been established, the next time this homeostatic deviation arises a neural impulse will at once emerge which will seek to re-activate the memory trace of the perception and to re-evoke the perception itself, that is to say, to re-establish the situation of the original satisfaction. An impulse of this kind is what we call a prediction; the re-appearance of the perception is confirmation of the prediction; and the shortest path to such confirmation is a path leading directly from the homeostatic deviation to a complete re-activation of the perception.

The reason this passage sounds familiar is because I have quoted it before, in a translation that was halfway between the two versions I have just provided (see p. 83). These new changes allow us to better recognize the deep similarity between Freud's concept of 'perceptual identity' and contemporary models of 'controlled hallucination'. But why stop there? Let's allow ourselves a little more latitude in our reconstruction.

Matthew Cobb was dismissive of Freud's 'Project for a Scientific Psychology', calling it a 'strange document' with no significance for our understanding of the brain.[10] Allan Hobson was positively rude about it, 'outing' Freud as a crypto-biologist whose theories relied upon antiquated neurophysiology: unfamiliar with central inhibition in the nervous system, his mental apparatus (according to Hobson) functioned by pumping a hypothetical nervous fluid called Q through a set of interconnected pipes – like the hydraulic puppets that so impressed Descartes in the royal gardens of Saint-Germain.

You can make this claim, if you must, but only if you focus on tiny details that Freud got wrong. If you focus instead on the much bigger picture that he got right, you will recognize, as Friston did (and Ostow before him), that the 'free energy' that drives Freud's mental apparatus is not fundamentally different from the uncertainty-reducing processes that govern the Free Energy Principle as we understand it today.

Here are the opening lines of Freud's 'Project', in Strachey's translation:

> The intention is to furnish a psychology that shall be a natural science: that is, to represent psychical processes as quantitatively determinate states of specifiable material particles, thus making those processes perspicuous and free from contradiction. Two principal ideas are involved: [1] What distinguishes activity from rest is to be regarded as Q, subject to the general laws of motion. (2) The neurones are to be taken as the material particles.[11]

I recently 're-translated' the passage as follows:

> The intention is to attempt, once more, to furnish a psychology that shall be a natural science; that is, to represent mental processes as quantitatively determinate states of specifiable physical elements, thus making those processes perspicuous and free from contradiction. Two principal ideas are involved: (1) What distinguishes activity from rest is to be regarded as F,* subject to the general laws of information.† (2) Neurons are to be taken as the physical elements.[12]

---

* Variational free energy.
† Shannon (1948).

This was not in my capacity as editor of the *Revised Standard Edition* (that really would be throwing professional integrity to the winds). Rather, it was an attempt to follow the advice of Luria's collaborator, Karl Pribram, who was amazed at the depth of Freud's insights when the unpublished 'Project' first came to light in the 1950s. On the basis of this work, Pribram 'welcomed psychoanalysis back into the natural sciences', describing Freud's Project as a 'preface to contemporary cognitive theory and neuropsychology'.[13] He suggested, in several articles and a book, that a reintegration of Freud's psychoanalysis with contemporary neuroscience would greatly benefit both disciplines.[14] Twenty years later, the neurophysiologist and Nobel laureate Eric Kandel expressed similar sentiments, writing that 'psychoanalysis still represents the most coherent and intellectually satisfying view of the mind',[15] and calling for 'a new intellectual framework for psychiatry'[16] based on its integration with neuroscience.

Twenty more years later, I published an updated version. Pribram had called Freud's Project 'the Rosetta Stone of psychoanalysis and neuroscience', and Rosetta Stones are of course primarily of interest to translators. Rather than merely translating the German into English, however, I wanted to replace Freud's original functional concepts with functionally identical modern ones. The paper appeared in an interdisciplinary journal, accompanied by open peer commentaries written by psychoanalysts and neuroscientists who shared Pribram's aspirations for the future of mental science. Karl Friston's commentary was particularly encouraging.

> This is a remarkable achievement but not entirely unanticipated. [. . .] Given that Freud built upon the foundations laid by Helmholtz, the reunion of Freudian and Helmholtzian thinking on offer in the *New Project* should be of no surprise. Although the mathematical details may take a few years to tie down with precision and grace, I think all the heavy lifting has been accomplished with this (re)visionary monograph.[17]

Of course, there's a sense in which, when we want to make someone seem reasonable, we try to make it look like they agree with us – as if what we think is the truth. Yet some of Freud's writings are not so amenable to translation in this way; and where we disagree with him, or can't make sense of him, it might be we who are at fault.

In a beautiful and important paper titled 'Mourning and Melancholia' (1917), for example, Freud wrote that in some cases of depression, following the loss of an attachment object, 'the shadow of the object fell upon the ego'.[18] A *Schatten* can only be a shadow, but here we are dealing with metaphor. What kind of shadow is cast by a lost loved one? Is it your persisting memory trace of them as a lost object? Is it the object's presence experienced now only in the negative: by its absence? Is it the dark side of the object, its less-loved residue? Is it a partial eclipse of the subject? Whatever it means, it is poetry: a rearrangement of the alphabet of science. If psychoanalysis were *only* science, then Freud would have had no need to write like this.

At other times, though, he really does seem to get it wrong. If the penis is envied, then surely it is not because mammalian genital anatomy 'is destiny'[19] but rather because our inevitable social hierarchy has been arranged in a particular fashion – which can be changed. (In bonobo groups, for example, females typically dominate.) Another striking mistake was Freud's assertion that 'the id' – the repository of our drives – is unconscious. If 'the pleasure principle governs the passage of events in the id with despotic force',[20] as Freud asserted it did, then how can it be unconscious? What is the point of a pleasure that you don't feel? How can the Freud who asserted (correctly) that feelings are always conscious also claim that the pleasure principle governs anything unconsciously? The id and the unconscious are, clearly, different mental agencies.

His postulate of a 'death drive' was another egregious error.

His claim was that 'the aim of all life is death'.[21] Really? His evidence was the fact that pleasure-seeking has its limits; eventually we've had enough and just want to be left in peace. He was right to intuit, belatedly, that a deep motivating force within us lies 'beyond the pleasure principle': what he called the 'Nirvana principle'. This force, he recognized, seeks not pleasure but quiescence. Yet modern biology teaches us that this quiescence is homeostasis: in other words, satiation, the ideal state of life, which is anything but deathly. Pleasure informs us that we are heading in the right direction: *towards* quiescence.

And then there's sex. Most of the controversies surrounding Freud's theories can be traced back to a single problematic claim: that mental disorders of all kinds arise from failures to satisfy not just any emotional needs, but specifically *sexual* ones.

His grounds for making this claim were, in the first instance, empirical. The aim of the psychoanalytic technique was to track patients' symptoms back to the life events that occurred when the symptoms first appeared. This led him to a surprising discovery, as he saw it: neurotic disorders were always triggered by either (1) premature sexual experiences or (2) an unsatisfactory method of obtaining sexual satisfaction. Moreover, he claimed that these two causes produced different types of neurosis, which he called '*psychoneuroses*' and '*actual* neuroses', respectively. According to the young Freud, psychoneuroses arise from past (i.e., remembered, but repressed) sexual abuse, while actual neuroses arise from current sexual practices. The term 'actual' means pertaining to ongoing acts, such as the practice of coitus interruptus or excessive masturbation, i.e., something that the patient is doing now. The most common neurosis of this type was 'neurasthenia', nowadays called chronic fatigue syndrome or myalgic encephalomyelitis. So, Freud claimed that 'neurasthenia' was caused by unhealthy sexual practices, and that not only 'hysteria' but also major depressive disorder ('melancholia'), panic disorder ('anxiety neurosis'), obsessive-compulsive disorder ('obsessional neurosis') and many other mental disorders besides, were caused by prepubescent sexual experiences.

These, Freud found, not infrequently involved abuse by members of his patients' own families. After two years of testing his theory, however, he realized that he was mistaken. The memories of childhood seductions that some of his patients produced during treatment turned out – on deeper investigation – to be false. One of the most striking instances was the childhood origin of his own neurosis. In Freud's famous 'self analysis' (conducted in the 1890s), he could find no link between his own – admittedly mild – neurotic symptoms and childhood sexual abuse. He did, however, recall obscure feelings of sexual arousal during childhood – for example, once when he observed *matrem nudam** at the age of four. From then onward, Freud concluded that psychoneuroses were caused not only by childhood sexual *events* but also – in many cases – by 'phantasies', with the implication that these were wishful confabulations. Bearing in mind that the false memories specifically involved childhood *sexual* experiences, Freud came to the conclusion that children were not only frequently the passive victims of sexual abuse at the hands of their parents and relatives, but also that they must possess sexual desires of their own.

This was even more shocking than his original suggestion that all neurotic disorders have a traumatic sexual origin. How odd, therefore, that Masson would later attribute Freud's retraction of his 'seduction theory' to cowardice. How ironic, also, in light of Popper's later criticisms, that Freud retracted the theory because he had *falsified* it. By widening the scope of explanatory factors to include not only objectively verifiable events but also subjective phantasies, however, he made it much more difficult to catch it out a second time.

To support his new conclusions, he drew attention to the

---

* 'My mother naked'. Freud described what he saw in this coy Latin way in a letter to Fliess, dated October 3 and 4, 1897. (He initially mistakenly dated the scene to age two and a half.)

everyday occurrence of erections in little boys (even in babies, for example while they are being bathed); to masturbation in children; to their common tendency to exhibit themselves; to their curiosity about what goes on in their parents' bedrooms, and so on. (It is easy to forget that one just *did not talk about such things in the 1890s*.) But Freud didn't stop there. He drew attention also to the fact that babies suckle at their mothers' breasts even when they are not hungry; that little children suck their thumbs, which cannot possibly satisfy nutritional needs; that they take pleasure in urinating and defaecating, sometimes even in withholding their faeces; that certain vigorous bodily movements cause them to squeal with delight; and so forth. In short, Freud pointed out that much of what children do is *seeking pleasure for its own sake*.

At this point, you might reasonably ask what these behaviours have got to do with sexuality. The answer brings us to the nub of the problem: Freud used the word 'sexual' in a much broader sense than the rest of us do. For him, 'sexual' was synonymous with 'pleasurable'.* To explain, he drew a distinction between two fundamental kinds of need (or 'drives'): self-preservative and libidinal ones. (*Libido* is Latin for 'desire'.) Satisfaction of the self-preservative drives keeps us alive; satisfaction of the libidinal ones gives us pleasure. On Freud's view, mere survival is not pleasurable in itself; self-preservation becomes pleasurable only to the extent that it is 'libidinized'. So, for example, sucking at a breast to satisfy the nutritional drive becomes pleasurable only to the extent that it satisfies a libidinal drive, too.

I say 'a' libidinal drive. Freud came to believe that there were many *components* of the libido. Sucking for its own sake satisfies the 'oral' part. But oral ways of obtaining pleasure are succeeded

---

* This is not a translation problem, but it is worth pointing out that the German word for 'pleasure', namely *Lust*, equally means 'desire'. Of course, it can also be translated as 'lust'. It is worth mentioning, too, that in Freud's times the German term for our 'sex' – in the sense of male vs female – was *Geschlecht*. *Sex* (the biological gender designation) was not current in German usage before the Second World War.

(according to Freud) during early development by 'anal' and then 'phallic' ways of doing so. These additional so-called component libidinal drives are expressed in some of the other childish pleasures mentioned previously, like defaecating ('anal' sexuality) and exhibiting oneself ('phallic' sexuality). According to Freud, these childish pleasures are superseded only at puberty by 'genital' sexuality; that is, by sexuality proper, in the sense that the rest of us use the term.

How might something like depression emerge from this conception? For Freud, what we nowadays call 'attachment' meant literally falling in love with one's mother. The loss of her as a 'love object' therefore implied loss of the person who previously satisfied your oral libidinal drive. All subsequent attachment bonds were just replacements for this primal one. Whenever you fall in love (regardless of your sex, gender identity or sexual orientation), the object of your affections is just standing in for your mother, who was your original oral fixation. The kind of sexual pleasure that you take in love has matured according to your stage of development, but the nature of the attachment is the same, and the loss of it will plunge you into despair. Depression, for Freud, is therefore just one of the mental apparatus's many responses to sexual frustration.

What to make of all this? Intellectual charity compels us to admit that there are forms of language in which we do seem to acknowledge a wider conception of sexuality than is usual in standard English. Roland Barthes and Susan Sontag taught us to think about art (in all its forms) in terms of the 'erotics' of aesthetic experience, its sensory and exploratory pleasures, broadly conceived. They were hardly operating independently of the Freudian tradition here, but here at least is a precedent, outside of strictly psychoanalytic discourse, for invoking a more capacious idea of the erotic.

And perhaps we can go further than that. Isn't there something in the idea that libidinous energies can infuse other areas of experience? Wasn't the whole modern advertising industry the result of Freud's nephew, Edward Bernays, realizing that seemingly innocent images and messages could tap into hidden wellsprings of sexual desire? Indeed, from a sufficiently godlike distance, isn't it clear that there really is something peculiar about sexuality? Our self-preservative drives preserve our measly selves, but genital sexuality is the main channel by which our biological commandment to *reproduce* makes itself felt. Isn't it? Isn't there a clear evolutionary sense in which, whatever we might take ourselves to be thinking or feeling, sex is what it's *really* about?

Well, I can tell you right now that there are many varieties of pleasure in the brain, and 'sexuality' and 'pleasure' are not synonymous. The brain circuitry for attachment bonding (the PANIC/GRIEF drive) – which produces, if not the most intense, then at least the most enduring pleasure in our affective repertoire – hardly overlaps with the circuitry for sexuality at all. The command neuromodulators for this form of attachment are mu opioids, whereas those for sexuality are the gonadal hormones oestrogen and testosterone, plus the peptides oxytocin and vasopressin. These two systems (for attachment and sexuality) can be triggered independently, in both animals and humans. There is little anatomical and chemical overlap between them. This is not to say that they can't operate simultaneously: they often do. Opioids, artificial forms of which include codeine, fentanyl and heroin, are of course highly addictive. Opioid-mediated attachment bonding, far from being a form of sexual interaction, might better be viewed as an addiction. (Freud, of course, thought masturbation was the 'primal addiction'.)[22]

I don't think there's any getting around the conclusion that Freud had this stuff seriously muddled. It is not that infantile sexuality doesn't exist, but that it is no longer tenable to describe every form of infantile (and adult) pleasure-seeking as the manifestations of one overarching 'libidinal' drive. Long before the discovery of dopamine in 1957, for example, Freud wrote:

> The neuroses, which can be derived only from disturbances of sexual life, show the closest clinical similarity to the phenomena of intoxication and abstinence that arise from the habitual use of toxic, pleasure-producing substances (alkaloids).[23]

He had personal knowledge of the effects of only one alkaloid, namely *cocaine*, which we now know is a potent *dopamine* booster. This is the command neuromodulator of the SEEKING drive, not the LUST drive. So, on the basis of what I have outlined so far, we can see that what Freud termed 'libido' decomposes into at least three drives: one for attachment bonding, another for something like exploratory interest (i.e., foraging), and yet another for good old sex.

At least half of the controversies surrounding Freud's libido theory can be traced back to his idiosyncratic conception of sexuality. It formed the basis of his quaint notion of the 'Oedipus complex'* (which he thought pivoted on infantile incestuous wishes); of his confused views about homosexuality (which he saw as a fixation at the 'pre-genital' stages of development); and of his sexist conception of 'penis envy' (which he saw as the inevitable outcome of so-called 'phallic' competitiveness; a competition that girls, with their smaller clitorises, can only lose). Perhaps less controversial now than it was when he originally proposed it, Freud also claimed that we are all 'bisexual' – although the way he used the term meant something similar to what we would nowadays call *non-binary* (in that, if there are such essences as maleness and femaleness, then everyone contains a mixture of both).

Alright, let's do this. Here is what we know today about the sexual circuitry of all mammalian brains, ours included. First, it is 'dimorphic', which means that it differs between typical males

---

* Freud was of the view that human beings are born with an innate predisposition to become sexually attracted first to their mother and then (in heterosexual girls and homosexual boys) to their father, coupled with equally innate murderous hatred of the parental rival who got there first. These erotic and destructive inclinations, according to Freud, are kept in check by an innate fear of castration (in boys) or the perceived fact of castration (in girls). For a modern conceptualization of this 'complex', see Solms (2022).

and typical females. ('Typical' here means the 68.2% of us who cluster around the centre of the bell curve depicted in Figure 1.) Second, we all possess both male and female sexual circuitry. So, Freud was right on that score. Third, the sexual circuit that dominates is determined by the relative quotas of testosterone and vasopressin (male-typical chemicals) versus oestrogen and oxytocin (female-typical chemicals) in the brain. Fourth, this divergence happens in utero at the end of the second trimester. Fifth, the extent of the divergence at that point in the maturation of each individual brain is determined by the levels of circulating testosterone and aromatase – the latter being an enzyme that converts testosterone into oestrogen, which, bizarrely, masculinizes the brain.* Sixth, importantly, this process occurs independently of the masculinization of the rest of the body. The latter process takes place much earlier (during the first trimester) and the extent to which it does so is determined by the levels of circulating testosterone and 5-alpha reductase – the latter being an enzyme that converts testosterone into dihydrotestosterone. Seventh, the level of circulating testosterone at steps five and six is determined by whether you have (functioning) testicles or not, which in turn is determined by whether the 23rd pair of chromosomes is XY or not.

In summary, it's complicated; which means that there may be many a slip between cup and lip. In 2016, I delivered the keynote address at a conference titled 'Transsexuality: Exploring a Challenge for Society at the Intersection of Theology and Neuroscience'. The conference was held at the Johann Wolfgang Goethe University in Frankfurt, but it was sponsored by the Lutheran Church – a representative of which, when he invited me, explained bluntly: 'We would like you to tell us whether God makes trans people the way they are, as this should determine our policy'. My answer was as simple as his question: 'Yes, if God makes people, he makes

---

* Why 'masculinize'? Because the default design of the mammal brain and body is female (but feminization is an active process too; it requires *suppression* of the masculinization process).

people like that'. This doesn't mean that *all* transgender people are literally born in the wrong bodies; but it certainly happens.

If masculine and feminine gender identity don't coincide with masculine and feminine sexual anatomy, and they are mixed in all of us, then what do 'masculine' and 'feminine' denote, really? Freud suggested 'active' and 'passive', which surely can't be right.

In pursuit of something more suitable, it may be helpful to review how current mental science finds that the male-typical brain differs from the female-typical one. First, it is bigger. Second, its corpus callosum is relatively smaller. Third, the interstitial nucleus of the anterior hypothalamus number three (mercifully abbreviated to INAH-3) is much bigger, though not (on average) in male-to-female transgender people or, interestingly, in homosexual men; gender identity and sexual orientation are certainly not the same thing, but there is some overlap between them when it comes to brain anatomy.[24]

What about behaviour? How does the male mammal differ from the female? Here our knowledge is fuzzier, but what can be said with confidence is that the male is typically more aggressive and engages in more rough-and-tumble play, whereas the female typically is more nurturant and more risk averse. These differences are not attributable to culture: I am speaking about mammals in general, and the differences appear to hold for every mammal species that has so far been studied.

I will end this brief survey of what we know about the innate sexual drive with two observations that apply equally to males and females, and to everyone in between. First, some relatively simple sexual actions are inborn – such as lordosis (exposing the anogenital area for penetration), mounting, intromission and pelvic thrusting. These are what we call 'instinctual predictions' as to how to satisfy your sexual drive. All the rest – i.e., how to get the individuals that you actually want to have sex with to agree to it – you have to learn from experience. That is a lot to learn. Second, sexual acts are motivated primarily not by the need to reproduce but rather by the fact that they *feel* good. Actually, most times when we have sex we are hoping not to reproduce, and many of the ways in which we do it cannot possibly produce a baby. This alone explains why we indulge in such a wide variety of sexual behaviours: we do whatever works for us, and then we automatize it.*

To come back to the most important point, Freud was plainly wrong when he said that all pleasures are sexual. I have described the sexual drive and differentiated it – and its underlying anatomy and chemistry – from opioid-mediated attachment and from the dopamine-mediated exploratory drive. Shortly I will introduce you to four more drives, and you will see that they, too, are not 'components' of sexuality.

The second most important point is that we are, nevertheless, motivated by pleasure for its own sake. This applies to every kind of pleasure, not only to sexuality. We don't become attached to our mother because we know, at six months or less, that we need her physical presence for purposes of nourishment, thermoregulation, protection from predators, and the like; instead, we attach because her presence *feels good*. Why does it feel good? Much the same reason chocolate tastes good: sweet things have high glucose content, so, on average, the ancestral mammals that liked sweet things survived and reproduced more frequently than those that did not. Therefore, their offspring like chocolate. The point is that we have no direct access to the reasons we like the things that we do: our preferences were given blindly, either by natural selection or by nondeclarative automatization. So, the real causes of (much of) our behaviour are *unconscious* – apart from the feelings. And that is what Freud said.

His view of sexuality is therefore both vindicated and corrected by current neurobiology. The correction boils down to this: many of the pleasures that Freud called 'sexual' are best called something else. Everything else that he got wrong about sexuality is detail, which flows from this singular error. What Freud said about

---

* I might add that this fact alone (which generalizes to all the drives) demonstrates that it is essential for biologists to take account of subjective variables if we are going to explain behaviour.

sexuality otherwise was pretty much valid, even some of the more counterintuitive things he said, such as that we are all 'bisexual' (non-binary) to varying degrees, and that we indulge in a wide variety of sexual behaviours because we are motivated subjectively by feelings rather than by rational, deliberative thinking.

In short, he was much more enlightened on sexual matters than he is given credit for. In the *Revised Standard Edition*, I have tried to offset the accusation of bigotry and homophobia by including some of Freud's writings that were overlooked previously, such as this letter, which he wrote (in English) to an American who asked him to 'cure' her son's homosexuality – although she couldn't quite bring herself to use the word:

Dear Mrs ——
 I gather from your letter that your son is a homosexual. I am most impressed by the fact that you do not mention this term yourself in your information about him. May I question you, why you avoid it? Homosexuality is assuredly no advantage, but it is nothing to be ashamed of, no vice, no degradation, it cannot be classified as an illness; we consider it to be a variation of the sexual function [. . .] Many highly respectable individuals of ancient and modern times have been homosexuals, several of the greatest men among them (Plato, Michelangelo, Leonardo da Vinci, etc.). It is a great injustice to persecute homosexuality as a crime, and cruelty too. [. . .] By asking me if I can help, you mean, I suppose, if I can abolish homosexuality and make normal heterosexuality take its place. The answer is, in a general way, we cannot promise to achieve it. [. . .] What analysis can do for your son runs in a different line. If he is unhappy, neurotic, torn by conflicts, inhibited in his social life, analysis may bring him harmony, peace of mind, full efficiency, whether he remains a homosexual or gets changed. [. . .]
 Sincerely yours with kind wishes,
 Freud[25]

This was written 39 years before the American Psychiatric Association removed homosexuality from its diagnostic manual, where it had been listed as a 'sociopathic personality disorder'. Sociopathy is defined as 'a mental health condition in which a person consistently shows no regard for right and wrong and ignores the rights and feelings of others'. (This disorder no longer exists in the DSM, but the closely related 'antisocial personality disorder' does.) Even when writing from deep confusion – caused by his belief that homosexuality was 'pregenital' – Freud was more on the money than his opponents. He was a decent human being with a profound sense of what matters, which seems to have guided him safely past many of the prejudices of his time and the partial detritus of his own theories alike. As a truth-loving scientist, he also left room for doubt, and for future advances in knowledge:

> I cannot discuss here whether each and every organ pleasure should be called a sexual one or whether, alongside of the sexual one, there is another which does not deserve to be so called. I know too little about organ pleasure and its determinants; and, in view of the retrospective character of analysis in general, I cannot feel surprised if at the very end I arrive at what are for the time being indefinable factors.[26]

So much for sexuality. And so much for the notion of a single pleasure-producing or pleasure-seeking drive. To the extent that the mind is a product of evolution, it naturally responds to certain overarching imperatives, among which the requirements of reproduction do stand out as being both unusually crucial and complex. Without that, the show comes to an end. But before you can reproduce, you must survive. Accordingly, the picture of the drives that has emerged in the past few decades of affective neuroscience research accords pretty well with what common sense might lead you to expect: we want sex, but also lots of other things that aren't sex.

There are many different pleasures that motivate us to pursue our wants and needs, and many unpleasures that motivate us to self-correct when we are drifting away from where we need to be. In modern neuroscience we generally call these feelings 'affects', though there are controversies here to which I will try to do justice below. Strangely, these too may be regarded as translation issues.

Each affect has its own distinct circuitry, which you can futz about with given a bone saw, an electrode and a strong stomach. (This was, in essence, how Jaak Panksepp and his colleagues mapped them out in the brains of such evolutionary near relations as monkeys, dogs, rats and even birds.) Each circuit exists to trigger a sequence of actions that resolves a need. These needs can be quite basic, in every sense: you feel the need to eat, or to empty your bowels, or to remove your hand from the hotplate. You relieve these felt urgencies as best you can within the constraints of the situation, which might, alongside bodily components, eventually come to include things like expected standards of behaviour, concealed threats, or the overall social impression that you are trying to give. As anyone who has potty-trained a child knows (or as anyone who has been a child knows), even the elementary bodily cues can take some effort to master. I would go so far as to say that *learning from experience how to meet our biological needs is the basic task of mental development.*

The behaviours that our needs trigger when they go unmet often have a stereotypical – not to say automatic – quality. Who doesn't recognize the 'separation distress vocalizations' and 'search behaviours' (as Panksepp called them) of children who have lost their mothers? You can recognize the same things in rats and dogs and even birds. To be clear, this behaviour is *not* automatic in the sense of having been consolidated into nondeclarative memory. Memory does not take the wheel. Reflex and instinct do, as passed down by natural selection. But these innate 'predictions' are too simple and stereotyped to work straight out of the box, so they need to be *supplemented* by learning. In desperate cases, indeed, the feeling might be more or less all that we are aware of, the oppressive need blotting out everything else and jerking us about like a puppet. With experience, we gain a measure of control over ourselves, but we never get over needing things. No amount of self-mastery can do that.* And the control that we gain, we gradually automatize, to free up mental space for life's many remaining unsolved problems.

What, in fact, do we need? This is a deep question, which goes to the very definition of what it is to be well. It should also help us work out what really helps in cases of mental illness. We will do our best to address this issue in the next chapter. For now, let's just observe that there is circuitry in the brains of all mammals, ourselves included, which appears to make us pursue much subtler objectives than eating, defaecating and so on. Panksepp called these objectives 'emotional' needs, as opposed to bodily ones. The sex drive is one of them, but it is by no means alone.

If any single brain system deserves to be equated with Freud's overarching pleasure-seeking drive, it is the dopaminergic all-purpose 'desire' circuit. I said earlier that this was initially called the 'brain's reward' system, and that the neuroscientist Kent Berridge called it the 'wanting' system. Panksepp initially called it the 'curiosity/interest/expectancy' system. Today the most widely used term for it in affective neuroscience is SEEKING, in Panksepp's canonical capital letters. Patients in whom this dopamine circuit is damaged become apathetic, apparently devoid of motivation and initiative. In fact, they seem very depressed.

At a conference in Tucson, Arizona, in 2006, I was able to show a positron emission tomograph (a PET scan) of what the dynamics of arousal in the dreaming brain actually look like.[27] Seeing the mesocortical-mesolimbic dopamine circuit lit up in the depths of sleep went a long way towards convincing my neuroscientific colleagues of the ongoing viability of the 'wish-fulfilment' theory of dreams. During waking life, Panksepp observed, 'direct electrical stimulation along this pathway results in the most energized exploratory and search behaviours an animal is capable of exhibiting.'[28]

---

* Even the Buddha had to defaecate.

The principal goal of the SEEKING drive is not sex but novelty. The evolutionary reason that we enthusiastically explore the new and the unknown is, paradoxically, because they are dangerous – but also potentially rewarding. Engaging with the new, proactively, in our own time and on our own terms, reduces its risks and increases our mastery of the world. To be the best steam engines we can be, we strive not to be caught out by the unexpected.

We have also met the attachment (PANIC/GRIEF) drive, which makes all mammals bond with their mothers for as long as they need to be suckled. In humans it remains active throughout our lives, creating the possibility of many profound bonds, of love and connection, or of pathological dependency, as the cards we are dealt dictate. When this drive to attachment is frustrated, we have a feeling of abandonment, also known as separation distress. We see this sequence of impulses play out in depressed patients: they protest initially and then they give up, the lost animal shifting strategy to conserve resources even as its chances of rescue dwindle, in a world filled with unknown dangers. In our own world this is experienced as depression, heartbreak, or (as both Freud and Panksepp separately suggested) grief. It remains active until attachment is re-established, either with the return of the original caregiver or through adequate replacements, which can be found only if you rebound. This happens when dopaminergic SEEKING, which is shut down in the 'grief' or 'despair' phase of PANIC/GRIEF, is reactivated.[29]

Completing our suite of affective circuits that clearly evolved, in the first instance, to guide us through the vagaries of reproduction and vulnerable infancy, it is worth noting that we also have hardwired impulses to *nurture*. Panksepp calls this the drive to CARE. Considering that we mammals are obliged to attach to our mothers, it is not surprising that there is a reciprocal biological impulse coming from the mother's side. It is also not surprising that this circuit is more sensitive in female-typical brains than male ones: it is modulated by oestrogen, oxytocin, prolactin and progesterone – all of which circulate at much higher levels (on average) in females than males, and especially during pregnancy.*

Like the others, this brain circuit triggers *instinctual* behaviours, in this case nurturing ones: we just 'know'† that when a baby cries the right thing to do is to pick it up, hold it close, rock it, make soothing 'motherese' sounds, and so on. Anyone who has raised a child knows also, though, that these stereotyped behaviours don't always get the job done. The rest of what you need to know must be learned, just as with the other drives. Yet the task of successfully rearing an infant is perhaps especially open-ended. What might it not demand of you? What *isn't* relevant to the welfare of a child? If you succeed, it feels wonderful in its own special ways (the pleasure of seeing our little ones thrive is boundless), but when you fail it feels commensurately rotten. One acute expression of being overwhelmed by the burden of care is post-partum depression.

It is important to recognize that, just as the PANIC/GRIEF variety of attachment generalizes beyond the mother/infant dyad to many other relationships, the same applies to CARE. We don't care only for our own offspring. The drive to nurture is not limited even to members of our own species: think of our love for pets. It is deeply reassuring to be reminded that not all biological drives are *self*-preservative; that altruistic needs lurk deep within us, too.

Another attachment drive (mentioned briefly in Chapter Four) is the need to be accepted as a member of the *group*, and to achieve status within it, since mammal societies are organized hierarchically. This is the task of the drive to PLAY. The instinctual behaviour associated with this drive is rough-and-tumble jousting: we do it, dogs do it, cats do it, squirrels do it; even dolphins do it, after their own fashion. There are two biological imperatives involved here.

---

* Astute readers might notice that there *is* some overlap, after all, between the CARE circuit and the female-typical LUST circuit.
† We don't really *know*, of course. The extent to which these inclinations are given blindly by nature is demonstrated by the fact that the great majority of us cradle babies to the left of our body midline, without ever realizing it, and without knowing why.

The first is revealed by the fact that, although children just love to play, most sessions end in tears. The one child says to the other: 'I'm not playing with you anymore; you're not being *fair*'. Studying how play breaks down (not only in humans) reveals something called the 60/40 rule: if the dominant playmate calls the shots too exclusively, there is no longer sufficient fun in the game for the submissive one. So, learning how to play teaches us to take turns – that is, to satisfy our emotional needs *in relation to the emotional needs of others* – and thereby, to build viable social hierarchies, where there is something in it for everybody.

The other rule of PLAY is the 'as-if' rule. If play fighting becomes real fighting then it is no longer PLAY, it is RAGE instead, perhaps with an admixture of FEAR. Likewise, if the cops-and-robbers game becomes too real – if you lock up your little brother and throw away the key – then you're not playing cops and robbers, you're locking up your brother. The doctor-doctor game allows you to undress your neighbour, but if you take it too far, it's not a game; it is LUST. So: the second major function of play (in addition to building viable social structures) is to enable us to *practise* how to meet our various emotional needs in a make-believe world, where the stakes are not as high as they are in reality.

People who fail to learn how to satisfy this drive tend to be overly concrete and unempathetic. They are asocial or even antisocial, and though commonly obsessed with status and rank, they cannot play the game. As a result, they lack the satisfaction they might otherwise have found in friendship, mutual and reciprocal relatedness, belonging and kinship, self-respect, and so on.

I have just mentioned the final two basic emotional needs: RAGE and FEAR. It is easy to understand the biological imperatives of RAGE. If someone stands between you and what you need – in effect preventing you from getting your share – then, unless you learn how to defend yourself, you are going to cop it. The homeostatic demand here (modulated mainly by a peptide called substance P) is felt as frustration, then as irritation, then anger, then fury. The instinctual response is 'affective attack': in other words, hit, kick and bite until the impeding object relents, or, if they don't, until you destroy them. Needless to say, this stereotyped response doesn't always work; so, as with all the other drives, we must learn from experience what else to do.

It is equally easy to understand the biological imperatives behind the FEAR drive. Here, the homeostatic set-point (where we need to be) is a state of safety. As soon as we sense danger, we feel fear, which, to be clear, is not the same as panic. In the case of panic, we search for the (separated) object, but in the case of fear, the instinctual response is the opposite: we freeze, or flee from the object. (This is why fear responds to benzodiazepines and panic doesn't; they have different brain chemistries.) There are several *innate* triggers of the FEAR circuit. Snakes and spiders are the best examples (even six-month-old babies startle when they see them), but the same applies to the objects of all common phobias. It seems that we are born with these phobias, then we must unlearn them.*

In addition, we must learn what *else* to fear, because there are many dangerous things in this world that natural selection could not have predicted – live electrical wires, for example. So, yet again, we must learn from experience. Fortunately, nondeclarative memory provides a particularly useful mechanism here; it's called 'single exposure learning'. Unlike attachment bonding – which requires you to learn who is a reliable caregiver over time – fear conditioning requires but a single exposure. Imagine what would happen if you had to touch the live wire again and again to ensure that it reliably produces a shock. Just as we saw in the case of other nondeclarative memory functions, this mechanism can be hijacked: that is how the symptoms of post-traumatic stress disorder (PTSD) arise. A single traumatic exposure to a terrifying stimulus (a gunshot, say) generalizes to all sudden loud noises, which makes you respond to them, too, as if your life were in danger.

---

* It is easy to see why fear of spiders, snakes, heights, the dark, etc., improves our chances of survival and reproductive success. The same, I dare say, applies to 'castration anxiety': those of our ancestors who feared damage to their penises are more likely to have reproduced than those who did not.

Are these seven emotions (LUST, PANIC/GRIEF, SEEKING, CARE, PLAY, RAGE and FEAR) all the basic ones we have, or might there be more? The answer depends mainly on how we classify them. For example, there is a body of opinion that disgust should be considered an emotional affect rather than a bodily one.[30] I am not sure that it matters, so long as we recognize that disgust exists; that it is an affective natural kind. What about other stuff we feel regularly, such as happiness? Is that one thing, a cocktail of things, or a myth? The answer here, too, depends on how you classify emotions. Panksepp used deep brain stimulation and chemical probes, and he came to the conclusion that 'happiness' can be decomposed into several more basic things. Paul Ekman, however, used facial expressions and concluded that it is a natural kind. In Panksepp's view, that is only because the happiness of SEEKING and of PLAY (for example) cannot be distinguished by their facial expressions – although their overall behavioural expressions are distinctive. Incidentally, which facial expression characterizes LUST or CARE? And who would deny that these are natural kinds of emotion?

We need also to consider the relationship between the natural kinds of emotion and our rich (human) vocabularies of emotional expression, both conceptual and behavioural. Lisa Feldman Barrett has observed, correctly, that there is a fair bit of cultural variation in this department.[31] Indeed, 'emotions for which there is no word in any other language' may have been a mainstay of cocktail-party discourse on the ontology of emotional life since the day that cocktails were invented.

Isn't this a problem for our account? On the contrary, when we think about what these brain systems are supposed to do, precisely what we would expect to see is variation in their expression, mediated by culture. If stereotyped behaviours were adequate to satisfy our needs, there would be nothing to learn. Barrett accepts that innate brain circuits and instinctual behaviours such as those I have described in this chapter do exist,[32] but she calls them 'motivated behaviours' rather than 'emotions' – partly on the grounds that we cannot know what animals feel, and partly on the grounds that animals lacking language cannot conceptualize their feelings in the ways we do. She hazards a guess that animals do feel something that she calls 'affect' rather than 'emotion': pleasure versus unpleasure and high versus low arousal. But that, it seems, is all.

Once again, we find ourselves wrestling with the slipperiness of words. Barrett starts with the culturally variable semantics and highly individualized shades of adult human emotions, and observes that these don't pick out anything well defined at the level of the cortex. From this, she concludes that emotions can't be natural kinds, and so they must be culturally constructed. From my point of view, I would say that this just demonstrates what is lost if you study the brain only from the psychological side of the microscope – a good thing for psychoanalysts to be cautious about.

Language, as Luria taught us, and Freud before him, is a complex psychological function. It must be analysed psychologically. The goal of such analysis is not to characterize the differences between cultures, interesting as that might be. It is to find the underlying component functions that are the true natural kinds at the level of the mental apparatus. Only then can we expect to make headway in identifying their anatomical and physiological correlates. This is, ultimately, a 'metapsychological' job. Getting it done will call for determined, imaginative and sympathetic co-operation between psychoanalysis and neuroscience, those two great nations still unfortunately divided by their common task.

It is relatively easy to satisfy our bodily needs: how to eat, drink, breathe, and so on. These needs generally involve inert substances, such as food, water and oxygen. Our emotional needs involve living subjects with minds of their own, which makes them far less predictable. What's more, our emotional needs frequently *conflict* with each other. When we are frustrated, for example, our instinct is to attack and destroy. When we are abandoned, we try desperately to regain loving care. What happens if both these needs are aroused by the same person? Well, whose mother never frustrated them? It is a real problem that, when she does so, our innate impulse is to attack her. (Anybody who has seen a baby whose need for sustenance or sleep or whatever is being frustrated knows what RAGE looks like.) This conflicts directly with PANIC/GRIEF; with our need to keep our caregiver's love forever. The typical outcome of this conflict is *guilt*, which is to say, inhibited rage, directed inwards rather than outwards: 'I am bad'.[33]

Another common conflict involves RAGE and FEAR. As I said, the instinctual response to frustration is to attack and destroy. But if we want to attack someone bigger than us (as the prohibiting parents of young children usually are) then hostility towards them is dangerous, arousing fear. The technical term for feelings of danger which arise from our own hostile impulses rather than objective external threats is *paranoia*.

It's remarkable how, though Freud didn't understand the drives in the way we do today, he still inferred from clinical observation the existence of conflicting inner priorities, and came to regard these tensions as pivotal in mental development. He had a habit, in fact, of reducing human mental conflict to slightly crude dichotomies: sexuality vs self-preservation; pleasure vs reality; drives vs civilization; etc. The ubiquitous childhood conflicts between RAGE on the one hand and PANIC/GRIEF and FEAR on the other that I have just described are the origin of what Freud called the 'superego' (actually Strachey called it that; Freud called it the *Überich*).

In his final conceptualization of the mind in conflict, Freud concluded that the 'ego' (*das Ich*) has three masters: the drives of the id (*das Es*), the constraints of reality, and the strictures of the superego. The latter agency (the superego) was assumed to be a natural kind: the inevitable residue not only of parental authority but also of genetic inheritance – the phylogenetic memory of a tyrannical 'primal father'. Neuropsychoanalytic research suggests otherwise: that the superego breaks down into several parts – an internalized object of RAGE, but also internalized objects of PANIC/GRIEF and FEAR, all of which conflict with one another and also with the rules of PLAY.*

The important thing is that it is not only difficult for us to learn realistic ways of satisfying each one of our emotional needs in their own right; it is even more difficult to reconcile these various needs with each other.

Romantic love is a commonplace example of the requirement to balance multiple emotional needs. Obviously, it involves lust; otherwise it wouldn't be *romantic*. But it also involves attachment (otherwise it wouldn't be *love*). And attachment is a two-way street, so it involves care, too. Negotiating who cares for whom, and more generally whose needs are prioritized – in other words, ensuring that emotional resources are distributed fairly – concerns the play drive. Play is implicated in power dynamics, and in ensuring that both partners have fun. When things go wrong in any of these respects, rage must be accommodated, since tolerating a certain amount of frustration is necessary in any successful relationship. And then there is novelty seeking: the attachment drive wants us to keep our partner's love forever, whereas the SEEKING drive is always on the lookout for *who else* is available. If you are going to have successful romantic relationships, you need to learn how to reconcile all these needs with each other.

And the same applies to the rest of life. The overarching task of mental development – and therefore a reasonable measure of mental health – is learning how to satisfy all seven of our basic emotional needs in an integrated way. That, alas, is far more difficult than deciding how to render technical German vocabulary in English.

---

* To be clear: the 'superego' is not an innate mental structure; it develops (almost inevitably) from the conflicting demands of the elementary drives. The same applies to the 'Oedipus complex' (see Solms, 2022).

The psychological manifestations of the basic emotional circuits that Panksepp identified were of course *observed* by Freud – from his end of the microscope – but he interpreted them differently. When he observed the addictive attachment of babies to their mothers, he interpreted it as oral sexuality. When he observed the unfettered rage of the human infant, he interpreted it as anal sexuality (which he sometimes called anal 'sadism'). When he observed the rivalries and jealousies of the nursery and the playground, he interpreted them as phallic sexuality. Today we call it PLAY. And lust, of course, Freud called genital sexuality. I could do a find-and-replace job on these terms, too, and Freud's drive theory would be essentially preserved.

One further problem would remain, however. Freud was of the view that the libido developed through these component drives in sequential stages – first oral, then anal, then phallic, and finally genital – whereas, in fact, they all are present from the get-go, even genital sexuality (recall those baby erections and the fact that infants masturbate).* The drives operate in parallel, but they display different *critical periods*. Thus, the baby must attach to its mother in the first six months of life. The frustrations of toilet training (and not only of toilet training) follow later. The need to find our place in the social hierarchy begins in the family but it makes much greater demands when we proceed to school. Genital sexuality makes unprecedented demands when we enter puberty, and this long period of latency is one possible reason that sexuality represents a weak link in our emotional make-up: if we've barely managed to cobble together a viable 'predictive model' to cope with the competing demands of the other emotional drives, the additional burden of adolescent sexuality can be the straw that

---

* Thus, whereas Freud conceptualized 'perversion' as fixation at a pregenital stage of libidinal development, it is more reasonable to think of paraphilic disorders (to use the DSM-5 nomenclature) in terms of unsuccessful integration of lust with the other, non-sexual drives, such as the drives to attach, to attack or to dominate.

breaks the camel's back.* There's no denying that it's difficult. One good consequence of Freud's excessive focus on sexuality may be that it corrected for an even more dangerous public disinclination to talk about it.

In the end, I decided to change only one major technical term in the *Revised Standard Edition*. Strachey erroneously translated *Trieb* as 'instinct'. Ironically, the person who is supposed to have 'falsely scientized' Freud was insufficiently familiar with the language of biology. A *Trieb* is a 'drive'; and an *Instinkt* is an 'instinct'. The two are very different: an instinct is an innate prediction about how to satisfy a drive – it is a *response* to a drive, not the drive itself, as anyone would know from a decent biology textbook.

One could update Freud's vocabulary to one's heart's content, and there are parts of his work that very much repay the effort. The feeling of having cracked his 'Project' is one of the great satisfactions of my long immersion in his work. Freud wrote the following at the time that he drafted it, in a letter to Fliess of October 20, 1895:

> In the course of a busy night [. . .] the barriers were suddenly raised, the veils fell away, and it was possible to see through from the details of the neuroses to the determinants of consciousness. Everything seemed to fit together, the gears were in mesh, the thing gave one the impression that it was really a machine and would soon run of itself.

---

* The loosened strictures that contemporary Western societies place on sexuality may be one reason why it is no longer as common a cause of psychopathology as it was in Freud's day. It's easy to forget just how absurdly regulated sexuality was in 19th-century Europe. Sex outside of marriage was absolutely forbidden in Catholic Vienna, for example, even in cases of widowhood, as indeed was contraception. (Freud was a fierce campaigner for 'marriage law reform', as some new material in the *Revised Standard Edition* demonstrates.)

Soon after, however, he realized that the gears were not in mesh after all, and the thing had not completely fitted together. He then abandoned the Project. When I resurrected it in 2020 – and, drawing upon more than a century of progress in neuroscience, hopefully completed at least a rough outline of it – I remembered Freud's poignant remark: 'the thing gave one the impression that it was really a machine and would soon run of itself'.

No machine can run forever without repairs and replacements; entropy makes sure of that. Freud is too capacious and transitional a thinker for his whole scheme to be factorized into modern terminology without remainder. The language that Strachey gave us may be imperfect, but it is now familiar and distinctively Freudian. We don't need to make Freud our contemporary to learn from him, and we don't need to rehabilitate every thought he had. If finding our own language for his best ideas helps us to separate them from his authority, to test them and develop them and make them our own, that's good enough for me. In any case, as Freud himself saw, the best ideas belong somewhere deeper than language.

CHAPTER SIX
Defence Mechanisms

> ANALYST: I am trying to understand. Why did you agree with me a few minutes ago that your arm is paralysed, and now you're not agreeing?
> PATIENT: Because you can't read my mind. In my mind's eye I can see that I am lifting my hand. But *you* can't see that.
> ANALYST: But what about with your physical eyes? If you look at your hand with your physical eyes, can't you see it is actually not lifting?
> PATIENT: [Nods.]
> ANALYST: So now which one do you think is right: what our actual eyes see or what our mind's eye sees?
> PATIENT: What your mind's eye sees.
> ANALYST: Does your mind's eye see something that is more real than what your physical eyes see?
> PATIENT: [Nods.]
> ANALYST: So that's why you believe you're not paralysed?
> PATIENT: [Nods.]
>
> — *From the author's clinical files*

Thomas W, in his late teens, was as depressed as anyone I have ever treated. His mother had been diagnosed with what turned out to be a particularly aggressive form of multiple sclerosis (MS) when he was a child. His father was a bus driver, who worked long hours, and who seemed to spend the rest of his time drunk. There was also a younger brother. They lived in a council apartment, which was effectively unfurnished, because the family were waiting to be moved to a more appropriate flat in light of the mother's condition. (She could no longer climb the stairs to the bedrooms.) For several years, as it turned out, they lived like that, out of boxes – which doubled as furniture – and they seemed to eat only junk food.

The father and brother were abusive. They called Thomas 'namby-pamby', because he was (in their view) excessively preoccupied with his mother's condition and with his own increasingly dark thoughts. Tom's father thought he needed to 'grow a pair'; and on one occasion, apparently to help him with this developmental task, he had hung him dangling over the railings of the upstairs balcony.

By the time Tom was referred to me, his mother was severely disabled in terms of both sensory and motor functioning. Nevertheless, she retained an optimistic outlook. (This is not unusual for a subset of MS patients. Charcot, the first to delineate the condition, called it 'morbid happiness'.)[1] She remained convinced that she, with the help of her devoted son, would continue to manage the household, even as she lost control over her bladder and bowels and became effectively bed-ridden (in a bed that had to be moved, single-handedly by Tom, to the downstairs sitting room).

Tom was referred to me by the neurologist who looked after his mother, not only because he was depressed but also because he was suffering panic attacks and hypochondriacal anxieties: he was increasingly worried that, like his mother, he had MS, which he did not. Instead, he had become psychologically fused with her. He spent every waking hour by her bedside – taking responsibility for her most intimate bodily functions and care. But his most disturbing symptom was that he was convinced, as he had been since childhood, that he and he alone would *cure* her. Initially, he spoke only of her deserving better care than she got from his father, and from the National Health Service. As his psychotherapy proceeded, however, it became clear to me that he believed he could – indeed must – literally cure her. His mother seemed to support this desperate conviction.

As she inexorably declined, however, and approached death,

Tom resolved that if he could not cure her, he would kill himself. She eventually died, having been admitted to hospital with pneumonia, three days after his 19th birthday.

I was informed of this event by the neurologist; so I sent an email to Tom, offering an emergency session. I needed to assess the risk of suicide and decide whether he should be admitted to the local psychiatric unit. Tom's reply was surprisingly breezy. He was doing fine, he assured me, and he would see me at the usual time, later that week. I therefore suggested that we have a brief telephone conversation, which we duly did. I asked Tom directly if he felt suicidal. He seemed surprised by the question, and reassured me, convincingly, that there was no risk of him harming himself.

On the Friday, when he arrived for his regular session, it became clear why he was surprised by my concern. He assured me that his mother was alive and well. In fact, if anything, things were looking up. I was confused. The doctor had informed me of her passing over the weekend, I said. 'How strange,' Tom replied. 'No, she's fine, thank you.' He continued: 'Actually, she's looking much better this week.' Bewildered, I apologized for the error, and picked my way through the remainder of the session trying to hold two possibilities in mind: either the neurologist had made a terrible mistake, which seemed hard to believe, or Thomas W had slipped into psychosis. I called his mother's doctor immediately after the session. She wasn't available, but an assistant assured me: Tom's mother had died six days ago.

I might have given the impression that the talking cure is something quite straightforward. You just note the patient's presenting complaint, take a history, get them to talk freely, help them to notice the pattern, then problematize it and link it with their symptoms so that they can act differently. Unfortunately, treatment is rarely so simple.

A man once unexpectedly turned up in my neuropsychology outpatient clinic, and for some reason I couldn't find the folder that usually comes with each referral. I therefore apologized and asked him (let's call him Johan T) to describe his complaint. 'I am not a patient,' he replied.

'Oh, that explains it then,' I said. 'So, please tell me, why are you here?'

'You know why I'm here.'

I didn't, and asked him to elaborate. He explained that he was a lawyer, and that he wanted me to stop 'the intervention'. He added that he had asked at the Health Professions Council of South Africa (HPCSA) whether it was ethical for a practitioner to deliver treatments without a patient's consent. They had told him it was not. Though he didn't accept my protest that I had no idea what intervention he could be talking about, at length he explained: I was planting women to seduce him. This was bad enough when it started, at work, but now that I was doing the same thing in his social environment the situation was untenable. I had to withdraw the women. He knew my intentions were good but, as the HPCSA had confirmed, I needed his approval to implement this treatment and – he repeated – I didn't have it. Unless I withdrew the seductive women forthwith, he was going to lodge a formal complaint.

He humoured my request for more information. It turned out that when he was a student at the University of Cape Town, he attended the Student Wellness Centre where he received counselling for 'relationship problems'. (*Romantic* relationship problems, he later clarified; it seemed to be a euphemism for sexual problems.) A short time after this counselling, the intervention began, first on campus and then at his place of work. He knew it was me who was behind it, because it required substantial resources, and I was head of the department of Psychology at the time. (Actually, I had nothing to do with the student counselling service.)

I respectfully explained that I could not do as he requested, because, despite appearances, I had nothing to do with this intervention. I accepted how it looked to him, from his point of view, but I could only say honestly that I had a different point of view. To my surprise, he was willing to hear me out, so I explained: what he was experiencing as these women's attempts to seduce him was his own sexual attraction to them. In fact he was 'projecting' his desire onto them, as Eglé Laufer taught me all those years ago.

'But how can what *they do* be a result of what *I feel*?' he retorted. I replied that it was a matter of what *he felt* they were doing, and explained using an example based on a recent experience: if you – and only you – know you are perspiring under your jacket, you might worry that the facial expression of the person you are sitting with shows disgust, when it shows nothing of the sort.

Again, to my surprise, he seemed to be open to my interpretation. If, hypothetically, what I said was true, he asked, what would my recommendation be: what should he do? I replied that my recommendation would be that he undergo psychotherapy, so that the inhibitions or anxieties that were causing his romantic difficulties could be dealt with, freeing him to have the erotic life that was currently eluding him. 'I knew it!' he said. 'You see! I told you: you are trying to force me to have sexual relations with those women.' With that he abruptly left my office, never to return, and lodged a complaint.*

This was an extreme example, but many patients are unwilling to enter psychotherapy. Some of them really are sent to us against their will. When parents send their children for analysis, for example, they don't necessarily come voluntarily. The same applies, even more so, when they send their rebellious and resentful adolescent kids. Similarly, in cases of anorexia nervosa or addiction, it tends not to be the patients who are worried so much as their parents and doctors. (It is tragic how many addicts believe that, unlike all other addicts, they have their habit under control; and when they come for treatment it is not to relinquish their addiction but rather to regain control over it.) In rarer cases, in countries where the courts offer psychotherapy as an alternative to incarceration – for domestic violence, sexual offences, and some other antisocial behaviours – patients are literally sentenced to

---

* After asking me to respond in writing, the HPCSA informed the complainant that his matter would not proceed to a formal hearing.

psychotherapy. In these cases, too, it is not primarily the patients who are suffering, but rather those around them.

This puts the analyst in a difficult position. Such patients are not willing collaborators in the process of working out where their suffering comes from, because they are not suffering. They might feel there's nothing wrong with them, or that the only thing they are struggling with is the unreasonableness of the authorities now subjecting them to the tedium of your company. The normal motivation for what we call a 'therapeutic alliance' is absent. Perhaps you have heard the joke: How many psychoanalysts does it take to change a lightbulb? One, but the lightbulb has to really want to change.

The term 'therapeutic alliance' reflects the fact that a psychoanalytical treatment requires trust. With patients who consciously (and for all one knows, correctly) believe that the therapist is working for their oppressors, it's hard to accept a suggestion that, for example, their eruptions of hostility reveal repressed predictions – 'transferences' – and not how they truly feel about their current predicament. And if the therapist actually is doing the bidding of the parents, say, instead of aligning themselves with the patient's own interests, some hostility may even be warranted. At the very least, this is bad professional practice (which is not to say it never happens).

In reality, it is true that patients do often prompt unhelpful emotional responses in their therapists, including anger. Standard practice is for the therapist to recognize these 'countertransference' reactions in themselves, then nip them in the bud, and use them to better understand what the patient is doing and feeling. Despite the obvious difficulties – and not to minimize the training and skill required – if an alliance is in place, both parties can typically navigate these choppy waters, and use the mutual understanding that such transference/countertransference enactments provide to good therapeutic effect. But as the joke warns: the patient must really want to change.

The ultimate motive in this regard is almost always their own suffering. You might think that, for a patient who isn't suffering, there can be no good reason for them to be in treatment in the first place. There are, however, two conditions in which we might subject a person to treatment against their will: if there is significant risk of them harming themselves or others, or if they are not mentally capable of judging their own best interests. This sounds like a Catch-22, but there are solid legal guidelines for determining risk-of-harm and mental competency, and, in most countries, the bar is set quite high. In any event, such unwilling patients are not normally referred for *psychoanalytical* treatment, for obvious reasons: it doesn't work if they don't want to talk.

These caveats, therefore, do not describe the kind of opposition that psychotherapists like me face on an everyday basis. The more usual problem is somewhat murkier and much more theoretically interesting. If a patient is neglecting some basic emotional need, they should obviously suffer from the feeling that announces it, just as surely as a lack of hydration would be felt as thirst – were it not for the existence of what Freud called *defence mechanisms*.

A remarkable fact about 'lesions of ideas' is that, rather like physical wounds, they often trigger a sort of protective swelling or scarring. Although, because this reaction is of a purely psychological kind, perhaps a better analogy would be one that involves *behaviour*: if you have a broken foot, you avoid walking on it, which is all well and good, but if the fracture is such that cure requires surgical re-setting of a bone, avoiding pain in the short term is not the best treatment in the long term.

Freud described it like this:

> Defensive processes are the psychical correlative of the flight reflex and perform the task of preventing the generation of unpleasure from internal sources. In fulfilling this task they serve mental events as an automatic regulation, which in the end, incidentally, turns out to be detrimental and has to be subjected to conscious thinking.[2]

Why do we protect predictions that fail to satisfy our emotional needs? It clearly doesn't stop us from using them – otherwise problems would never arise, and symptoms never present. Simply put, this is why. Poor predictions lead to unmet needs, which lead to bad feelings. Defences are deployed to drown out the feelings, even though the needs remain unmet. The bad feelings recur, and the defences are again deployed, more easily this time because practice makes perfect. The more deeply consolidated and automatic the defence becomes, the more chronically the need is unmet. In short, it's a feedback loop, which can in many cases swell in intensity until something snaps. In other cases, the defences are retained indefinitely, due to what Freud called 'gain from illness' (many advantages can accrue from the sick role).

In the case of Thomas W, defensive denial of his mother's death didn't satisfy his underlying need of her. The need would be met only if *suffering* her loss eventually prompted him to find another, living person to attach to: someone who cared for him at least as much as he cared for her. Likewise in the case of Johan T: the defensive projection of his sexual desire didn't reverse the underlying frustration of the drive: that could be achieved only by him *facing* and then overcoming his sexual inhibitions and anxieties.

Of all the psychoanalytic notions that I have discussed in this book, defences might be the most commonsensical, the easiest to swallow, the hardest to dispute. 'Defence' means nothing more than *trying to avoid something*. Not even the most inveterate Freud-basher would deny that we have all sorts of ways of avoiding unpleasant realities: distractions, rationalizations, excuses, blaming others, burying our heads in the sand. As insights go, it is by now folk wisdom. We accept that all sorts of behaviours – drug or alcohol use, cutting, bulimia, anorexia – may be semi-wilful diversions from our real issues. We readily see innovations such as computer games, social media and internet pornography as crutches that help us avoid the feeling of not *really* meeting our emotional needs. Our propensity for running from problems and then pretending, even to ourselves, that we haven't, with baneful consequences, is a literary theme that traces back to the Akkadian

Epic of Gilgamesh (2nd or 3rd millennium BCE); that is, to the very dawn of literature.[3] You might therefore wonder whether it is fair to credit such a universally accepted idea to Freud alone.

My reply is that Freud crystallized the concept in three important ways, each of which displays a characteristic strength of his thought. First, he organized the variety of defences with great clarity. His catalogue of defence mechanisms was logical and elegant, if not exhaustive, and it has never been significantly improved upon. Second, he placed the concept in an explanatory context – the mental apparatus, conceived in functional terms – in which it appears almost inevitable. Finally, he had a kind of architectural vision for what subtle and varied phenomena could result from combinations of these simple elements. Another way of putting it is that he intuited how much of our mental lives they explain: how fundamental the defences are to our minds' way of working. They play a fundamental role in shaping what we call character.

Freud divided the defence mechanisms into three broad categories, running the gamut from bad to worse: 'neurotic', 'narcissistic' and 'psychotic'. All of us have defences of one sort or another; the accommodations we make to cover the inadequacies of our own ways of life to a certain extent *are* our personalities. But they aren't all equally successful. The more realistic a defence is – in the sense not of accurately representing reality, but of being compatible with it – the more reliably it can manage the troubling feelings that arise from the repressed predictions. The less realistic it is, the more likely it is to fail. This leads to mental troubles. When our defences against suffering are breached, we become emotionally unwell.

Freud called this the 'return of the repressed'. In fact, though, it is not the repressed prediction itself that returns to consciousness (that is impossible, since it is encased in the deepest, nondeclarative memory systems). What returns instead is the *feeling*: the unpleasant intimation that something is wrong, from which the defence had been protecting us.

The most realistic defences are the neurotic ones, of which the best-known example may be 'sublimation'. This means substituting the objects and aims of repressed predictions from their original childish forms to more socially acceptable ones. Take attraction to one's mother: if you replace her with a girlfriend or a husband, or with anyone else that is both socially acceptable and satisfies the drive, so what if they are a substitute for your mother?*

Other defences, such as 'introjection' or 'projection' (which are narcissistic) and 'disavowal' (a psychotic defence), are less easy to live with. In 'introjection', one denies the loss of an object by trying to become it. In a limited sense, this is what I did with Clifford Yorke (although I would claim that mine was a neurotic defence, since I *substituted* my longed-for connection with my father by a connection with Yorke). In a more acute way, this is what Thomas W did with his ailing mother: he *became* the mother by caring for her in place of her caring for him – with the cost that he developed hypochondriacal beliefs that he had MS. In 'projection', by contrast, one locates the source of one's suffering in the object instead of oneself. This is what Johan T did: he experienced his troublesome sexual drive as coming from the women that I had purportedly planted around him rather than from within himself.

'Disavowal' involves withdrawing from and thereby denying the part of reality that causes prediction error. Some problems seem too enormous to deny, and yet deny them some of us do. The clinical evidence is formidable. When Thomas W slipped into psychosis, he disavowed the unwelcome reality of his mother's death, and then, to quote Freud, a 'delusion is found applied like a patch over the place where originally a rent had appeared in the ego's relation to the external world'.[4] That is, he replaced the unacceptable fact of his mother's death with the delusion that she was not only alive but also doing rather well. And he clearly believed that this was true.

People often throw the words 'neurotic', 'narcissistic' and 'psychotic' around very loosely. In Freud's day, 'neurotic' covered

---

* What makes this manoeuvre neurotic? Well, according to Freud, we are all at least a little bit neurotic; there is no such thing as absolute mental health.

all the functional neurological disorders. However, as we have seen, he believed that only the *psycho*neuroses had a psychological aetiology; he thought that *actual* neuroses were physiological in origin – that they were caused by intoxication or withdrawal from (what he mistakenly took to be) sex hormones. 'Psychotic' has always denoted loss of contact with reality, as it still does, and it was generally recognized as being either psychological or physiological in origin, as it still is. The term 'narcissistic' was introduced by Paul Näcke and Havelock Ellis at the turn of the 19th century, but it had a very limited meaning: it referred only to 'auto-erotic' behaviours like masturbation. It was Freud who gave it the wider meaning it has nowadays: an organization of the personality around various forms of self-love.[5]

In psychiatry today, the term 'neurotic' has been dropped from our official diagnostic categories, and 'narcissistic' is used only with reference to personality disorder. The term 'psychotic' is used in both psychiatry and neurology. The overarching term that Freud used in relation to all these disorders – namely that they were 'neuropsychoses of *defence*'[6] – is used only by psychoanalysts and psychoanalytic therapists. If biological psychiatrists were to use the term 'defence', of course, that might imply their endorsement of Freud's whole psychodynamic model: a dangerous thought.

Some years ago, the neurologist V. S. Ramachandran sent a letter about me to *Scientific American*. 'I applaud Solms's efforts to link the findings of modern neuroscience with some of Freud's intuitive hunches,' he wrote. 'The so-called Freudian defence mechanisms – such as rationalization, denial, repression and reaction formation – are a vital and very real part of our mental life, although most neuroscientists are in denial about this.'[7]

A good joke: the denial of denial. Yet it remains the case that neuroscience hasn't done much with the concept. That's a shame, because there's surely a great deal to discover.

Ramachandran, as it happens, wrote his letter after observing a strange issue in one of his own patients. He was caring for a woman after a stroke in her brain's right hemisphere paralysed the left side of her body.[8] The thing was, she denied that she was paralysed. She insisted, quite vigorously, that she could move her arm perfectly well. Yet the arm did not move. Diagnosis: anosognosia, a neurological condition in which the patient is unaware of their neurological condition.

When the neurologist and psychoanalyst Edwin Weinstein first suggested that it might be a product of defensive denial,[9] the (generally accepted) counterargument was that if that were so, then denial would occur equally with left- and right-sided paralysis; but it occurs only with the former, so it must have something to do with the *location* of the brain damage.[10] Ergo: a right-hemispheric cognitive deficit, not a psychodynamic defence.

That might have been the end of the story. However, being a doctor with an experimental bent, Ramchandran had the idea of artificially jolting his patient's attention to her left side using a method called caloric stimulation. Cold water is squirted into the (left) inner ear, triggering a distinctive reflex pattern of eye movements. This is startling but painless, harmless, and, crucially, it isn't able to reverse any underlying tissue damage. Nevertheless, the patient not only immediately confessed to her paralysis; she revealed that she had known it all along, by accurately dating its duration. When the stimulation wore off, she went back to denying it. In fact, she recalled everything that had happened in her conversation with Ramachandran during the caloric stimulation (even the design of the necktie he was wearing), with the singular exception of the part where she admitted to being paralysed.

This is very suggestive. A condition that was assumed to be due to simple destruction of neural tissue – as it were, the deletion of the part of the brain that could acknowledge this aspect of reality – turned out to yield to an intervention that didn't alter the destroyed tissue in any way.

Ramachandran subsequently reported that it was possible to get such patients to acknowledge their disability by injecting a placebo into their paralysed arm and saying that it would cause only *temporary* immobility. This was confirmed when he tested the hypothesis.[11] (Good old falsifiability again.) My own research group and others have since reported a raft of experiments which demonstrate the same thing.[12] Crucially, we have shown in various ways that anosognosic patients have implicit (nondeclarative) knowledge of their paralyses. Moreover, we have demonstrated that it is possible to overcome the denial not only by caloric stimulation, as Ramachandran did, but also by forcing these patients to observe themselves *objectively* – replacing their usual subjective view, using mirrors and video-recordings to show their paralysed behaviour from an outside perspective.

So, why does anosognosia occur only with right-hemisphere damage? The answer is that we are not born with an understanding of how three-dimensional space works; we must learn it. It is difficult to learn how to put yourself in somebody else's shoes; to see yourself from the outside, objectively. This is not only difficult cognitively; it is also difficult emotionally. When this hard-won knowledge is lost with right-sided brain damage (as it is, since the right hemisphere is specialized for spatial cognition), patients revert to *wishful* ways of construing spatial relations. They either 'introject' the now-lost functional limb or they 'project' the currently paralysed one. In the latter case, right-hemisphere patients *do* acknowledge that the arm is paralysed, but they claim it belongs to somebody else.*

Once again, we are dealing with the 'idea' of an arm, rather than with its concrete neural topology. In this sense, anosognosia (defensive rejection of paralysis) seems to be the obverse of hysterical paralysis (defensive adoption of paralysis) – the very condition that prompted Freud to start formulating psychoanalytic explanations in the first place.

There is something uncanny about these conditions, in a sense that Freud would endorse. When you can switch aspects of

---

* This condition is called somatoparaphrenia. It takes various forms, including 'supranumerary limbs', in which the patient says: 'Yes, that left arm is paralysed, but my other left arm is not.'

a person's sense of reality on and off like a light, it does feel as though you are engaging with them no longer as a living 'I' but as something inanimate – a mechanism. The effective interventions in these conditions are much closer in spirit to hypnotic suggestion than to a direct hotwiring of the brain's anatomical circuitry, and yet there is still something decidedly mechanistic about them. In such cases, the mind shows us its workings. Ramachandran himself concluded that anosognosia must be psychodynamic. If this is so, it can only imply that the *brain* utilizes psychodynamic mechanisms, such as, in this case, the mechanisms of defence.

There are none so blind as those who will not see. Ramachandran was willing to look, and when he did, he saw the obvious. As Freud put it, many others 'repeat in their resistance the classical manoeuvre of not looking through the microscope so as to avoid seeing what they had denied'.[13]

Where does all this leave the psychoanalyst? We want to dig out the faulty prediction that is causing our patient all their trouble, but our progress is opposed at every turn by a barrage of resistance.

Faced with a well-defended position, before trying to analyse the transference, one must reconnoitre the fortifications. Unlike repressed predictions, which are always aimed (albeit badly) at meeting an underlying need, defences arise to blot out the bad feelings caused by the inadequacy of the prediction.[14] They are an exercise in *avoidance*. This makes it harder to see what the need was. Therefore, defence analysis takes the form: 'Can you see that you are doing *this* in order not to feel *that*?'

To illustrate the difference between repression and defence: In the case of Thomas W, the repressed prediction was: 'I shall make mother better'. If his childish plan had succeeded, Tom would have gained a functioning caregiver (i.e., he really would have met the underlying need). The defence, by contrast, took the form: 'Mother is still alive'. This false belief didn't involve any plan of action; all it achieved was avoidance of an unwelcome truth causing a feeling of profound loss. Repressed predictions may not be realistic, but they are the best (or the least bad) plans of action that a small child can muster. Then they become automatized. Defences are less deeply seated: they are emergency measures; mopping-up exercises.

What comes to our aid when confronted by defences is the fact that, by their very nature, they tend to falter or fail. So, we use the fleeting moments when our patients' defences fail them – when the underlying suffering breaks through – as the starting point for our analysis. These sudden moments of vulnerability, horrible as they are for the patient, become a foundation of the treatment. They are moments of truth, to which both patient and analyst can refer back whenever defensive manoeuvres muddy the waters again.

In Tom's case, he was still claiming that his mother was alive and well in our next appointment, but his mood was more downcast. Some 15 minutes into the session, his face crumpled, and he sobbed into his hands: 'She's alive.' He remained like that, face in hands, for the next minute or so. I said: 'This overwhelmed feeling is what you're avoiding by telling yourself that she's still alive; but the feeling tells us that she is not. So, we must find a better way of dealing with your new situation.'

An unmet emotional need, such as the need for mothering, causes a constant trickle of bad feelings into the mind. The child desperately searches for a solution to the problem (for example, making mother better). Since the problem proves insoluble, the child eventually stops working on it: using a false prediction – a wish – he pushes it out of his thoughts as though it *were* solved. The bad feeling remains, but at least the child can focus on more tractable problems instead. If, for whatever reason, the original need now makes renewed demands (through permanent loss of the mother, for example), it proves difficult to overwrite the false prediction, which has become deeply consolidated. By comparison it takes little effort, in the short term at least, to simply avoid the difficulty and drown out the resurgent feeling.

And what are bad feelings? Well, from the neurophysiological perspective, they are the subjective result of the activation in the brain of various neuromodulatory chemicals. These chemicals, like psychoactive drugs, adjust how the brain and the body function in quite general ways. They tamper with your heart-rate, the speed of your reflexes, the ways that you form or access memories, and so on. From the subjective perspective, they tell you whether what you are doing is succeeding or not. The organism's responses to being 'on' these chemicals evolved to help it better deal with certain classes of existential threat, a different kind of survival situation for each of the main chemical cocktails. But where you aren't really dealing with such a threat, or where you are no longer at its mercy – where your brain is always in the wrong gear for the contexts in which you actually find yourself – you are what we might call *poorly adjusted*. Both your feelings and some of the deep-seated predictions that cause them are ill-suited for your present reality. What happens then?

In the ancestral environment, presumably you might have died quite soon. (Or rather, people like you will have died sooner and therefore reproduced less on average.) How else would the affective circuits have evolved? Why else would the mental apparatus register certain emotional relations as biological needs, similar in kind to such homeostatic necessities as food and air? In our current world, however, notwithstanding stories about deaths from a broken heart, people tend not to die of being afraid or angry all the time – or anyway, not quickly.

It is one of the ambiguous blessings of civilization that there is, as it were, no limiting factor on how long our emotional needs can go unmet. And so we can spend our lives under the intoxicating influence of contextually inappropriate emotions. This, not to put too fine a point on it, is the psychoanalytic account of what it is to be mentally ill. When something goes wrong with the mind, says Freud, it's this.

There is now a popular-psychology-level awareness of how something of this sort might explain the relationship between emotional disorders and that peculiarly ubiquitous 21st-century diagnosis of everything, trauma. In the popular conception, just about any unpleasant event (including mere verbal slights) can be 'traumatic'. I find it more helpful to think of traumatic situations as events for which you have no preparation at all. Here, it is not a matter of bad predictions so much as *no* predictions. That – the helplessness of it – is what makes such situations traumatic. Whereas repressed predictions are executed unconsciously, *no* predictions produce a state of heightened consciousness (of hyper-uncertainty). The whole scene enters awareness with great sensory clarity, charged with ambiguous significance. This is why PTSD (which follows real trauma only) is characterized by flashbacks: we literally re-live the traumatic moment, even in our dreams.

Yet PTSD involves more than this. It implicates also the mechanism of single-exposure fear conditioning, which I have described already. Remarkably, something similar seems to happen with the sex drive. For reasons that are still not entirely clear, one's first sexual experience casts a long shadow over one's subsequent sexual preferences. Victims of child sexual abuse not infrequently escape their tormenters only to find their way back into similarly abusive relationships – or become paedophiles themselves.* It's as if a die has been cast: sex means somebody abusing somebody. This equivalent of single-exposure learning in relation to the sexual drive might go some way towards explaining the lifelong consequences of childhood sexual encounters, as Freud surmised in the first place.

Be that as it may, all the common psychopathologies arise from failures to meet one or another of our ordinary emotional needs. So, just as a person who doesn't manage to switch off the fear circuit will suffer from post-traumatic stress disorder or phobia;

---

* I realize this sounds shocking, and I accept that many people will disagree, but the evidence is quite compelling (see for example Drury, Elbert & DeLisi, 2019; Freund, Watson & Dickey, 1990).

a person who doesn't satisfy the attachment drive will suffer from major depression or panic disorder, or borderline personality disorder or something else of that kind; a person who doesn't satisfy the exploratory drive will suffer from mania or attention deficit hyperactivity disorder (ADHD) or something similar;* a person who doesn't satisfy the aggressive drive will suffer from 'anger management' problems, and so on.

Perhaps you feel a certain doubt that this can really be all there is to mental illness. Surely medical science documents and treats conditions that are far too strange, too extreme in their severity to be explained as the simple result of *a chronically unsatisfied emotional need*. What about the terrifying hallucinations and delusions of schizophrenia? What of the seemingly barren expanses of autism, where even language fails to take root? One wants to say that these are genuine diseases, not just difficulties of emotional adjustment. They are problems to which the proper response is *medical* treatment, the kind of treatment that only real doctors can provide. In short, they must be problems for *psychiatry*: medicine's own medicine of the mind.

It's time, I suggest, to take a history.

When Freud studied medicine at the University of Vienna, his professor of psychiatry was Theodor Meynert, author of a famous textbook titled, simply, *Psychiatry* (1884). In its preface, Meynert wrote:

---

* What does it mean to satisfy a drive that is always looking for the next thing? In short, it means what The Rolling Stones song taught us: 'You can't always get what you want'. The Bible says the opposite: 'Seek, and you shall find', but that is (unfortunately) not true; sometimes we seek and we do not find. So, learning how to *really* satisfy the SEEKING drive is learning a better prediction than the biblical one; learning to curb your enthusiasms, to accept life's limitations. Kleinians call this 'the depressive position'.

> The reader will find no other definition of 'Psychiatry' in this book but the one given on the title page: *Clinical Treatise on Diseases of the Fore-Brain.*[15]

What sort of diseases? Meynert's answer was surprisingly specific: the purview of psychiatry was cases of cerebral vasomotor dysfunction. His theory was that when a part of the brain was activated by an emotion or a thought, life-giving blood was redistributed to the active part and away from an inhibited part. This redistribution would cause hyperaemia in the active region and vasoconstriction in the inhibited region. On this general basis, Meynert attributed schizophrenia to microvascular abnormalities in the cerebral cortex and hysteria to changes in blood-flow through the choroidal artery. Whatever the trouble, blood was the culprit.

The quotation from Meynert's *Psychiatry* continues:

> The historical term for psychiatry, i.e., 'treatment of the soul',* implies more than we can accomplish, and transcends the bounds of accurate scientific investigation.

The German word for 'mind' is *Seele*, which can also be translated as 'soul'. *Psyche* is a synonym for *Seele*. So, 'psychiatry' implies 'treatment of the soul'. This implication embarrassed Meynert – he thought that the very word denoted something that inhabited a different dimension from the physical body, a figment in a spectral realm floating alongside the solid everyday one. He was therefore determined to establish psychiatry on an entirely materialist footing, one that excluded the psyche. In this way, psychiatry lost its mind.

The trouble was, all the mental illnesses for which material causes could be established were allocated to a different medical

---

* The term psychiatry (φυχιατρική) comes from the Greek φυχή (psychē: 'soul or mind') and ιατρός (iatros: 'healer'). It was coined by Johann Reil in 1808.

department. 'Diseases of the forebrain', in the narrow sense that Meynert used the term, were the preserve of neurology, not of psychiatry. A century and a half ago, these two 'nervous' specialities first diverged from the broader field of *internal medicine*, that is, the study of diseases that occur inside the body, such that we must infer their causal mechanisms from external signs. The diseases that occurred inside the part of the body known as the brain were deemed sufficiently complex and numerous to deserve a speciality or two of their own.

There is a standard procedure in internal medicine: clinico-anatomical correlation. In the 18th century, doctors observed that patients who suffered from chest pains (upon exertion) during life were regularly found at autopsy to have clogged or narrowed coronary arteries. On this basis, when they subsequently encountered new cases of chest-pain-upon-exertion, they inferred that the underlying cause was a narrowing of the arteries, then treated the patient accordingly, even though they were unable in those days to inspect the state of their patients' cardiovascular system. This was the essence of internal medicine.

In the 19th century, pioneering physicians set out to do the same for diseases of the nervous system. That is how Jean-Martin Charcot founded the discipline of neurology: he correlated the outward manifestations of brain and spine disorders with their underlying pathological anatomy, which laid the foundations for a scientific, cause-and-effect understanding of the *mechanism* of each syndrome. This in turn pointed the way to cures. Multiple sclerosis (the disease that afflicted Thomas W's mother) was one of the many diseases that Charcot thus identified, enabling neurologists to make this diagnosis in an era when it was impossible to inspect the health of the living brain and spinal cord.

Why didn't 19th-century *psychiatrists* do the same? Perhaps you have already guessed. When patients with symptoms and signs such as those that we now call major depression came to autopsy, no anatomical pathology of the brain's tissues could be found. There appeared to be no underlying disease, and therefore nothing to correlate with all the peculiar mental symptoms and signs that the doctors wished to explain. The same applied to every neurosis and many psychoses. On this basis, the distinction between neurology and psychiatry was drawn: the former discipline was concerned with disorders of the *structure* of the nervous system, whereas the latter was concerned with disorders of its *function*. This distinction was (and still is) understood to mean that, although the anatomy of the brain is intact in psychiatric disorders, it is for some reason not functioning properly.

For what reason? As we have seen, Meynert hazarded a guess: for *physiological* reasons, specifically having to do with the flow of blood. That is what he took the word 'functional' to mean: physiological as opposed to anatomical. But the mechanisms that Meynert inferred were highly speculative, which is what prompted Freud to shift his allegiance to Charcot.

At the height of Charcot's fame as a neurologist, he urged serious scientific study of the neuroses. He was especially interested in the neurosis that was then called hysteria, in which patients displayed symptoms and signs of neurological disease but where no such disease process could be found at autopsy. Charcot's inclination was to approach this like any other problem in neurology: that is, to characterize its symptoms and signs and then wait for the pathologist's findings.

But hang on; isn't that precisely what is lacking in functional disorders: pathological findings? Yes indeed; so the emphasis here falls on the word *wait*. Charcot believed that hysteria was caused by a 'dynamic lesion' – in other words, by some kind of physiological abnormality in the activity of the brain that did not produce visible tissue damage. He expected that advances in medical technology would *one day* make it possible for doctors to visualize these 'dynamic' lesions in living patients in the same way that doctors of his own era could see anatomical lesions at autopsy with the naked eye. The only difference between Charcot and Meynert on this score, therefore, was that Meynert speculated about the specific nature of the pathophysiological mechanisms whereas Charcot elected to wait. In the meantime, he recommended that internists should carefully describe and classify the various functional disorders, in anticipation of a day when medical technology made it possible to explain them physiologically.

This is pretty much what they did. Modern psychiatry addresses the challenge of formalizing the diagnostic criteria (the 'syndromes') which constitute the multiplicity of psychiatric disorders, so that we can all agree upon what things like 'post-traumatic stress disorder' and 'schizophrenia' and 'attention deficit disorder' look like, clinically, in order to pave the way for a future understanding of their physiological causes. After all, unless researchers can agree upon the pattern of symptoms and signs that *constitute* syndromes like 'major depressive disorder' versus 'panic disorder' versus 'obsessive-compulsive disorder', and so on, it will never be possible to discover their different causal mechanisms, and develop appropriate treatments.

The crucial thing to note here is the assumption that the causal mechanisms would prove to be physiological. That is what makes this approach to psychiatry mindless. I don't want to be misunderstood. I'm not saying that *no* consideration is given to psychosocial factors in the authoritative conceptualizations and classifications used in psychiatry today; but these considerations are secondary ones, and they are still assumed for the most part to be mediated by physiological variables (so that, for example, 'stress' equals 'cortisol'). Likewise, not *all* mainstream psychiatric researchers are ruthlessly reductionistic. But if you take a look at the titles of the vast majority of scientific articles published in a recent issue of any of the major psychiatric journals, you will see what I mean.[16]

The enormous nosographic task recommended by Charcot has resulted in a big book called the *Diagnostic and Statistical Manual of Mental Disorders* (DSM). It was first published in 1952 by the American Psychiatric Association, and is now in its fifth edition, running to around 1,000 pages. It completely dominates modern psychiatric research and practice.*

---

* What I say here about the DSM applies equally to the World Health Organization's ICD (*International Classification of Diseases*), which is currently in its 11th edition.

The major classes of psychiatric disorder, as they are classified in it currently, are: neurodevelopmental disorders; schizophrenia spectrum and other psychotic disorders; bipolar and related disorders; depressive disorders; anxiety disorders; obsessive-compulsive and related disorders; trauma- and stressor-related disorders; dissociative disorders; somatic symptom and related disorders; feeding and eating disorders; elimination disorders; sleep–wake disorders; sexual dysfunctions; gender dysphoria; disruptive, impulse-control and conduct disorders; substance-related and addictive disorders; neurocognitive disorders; personality disorders; paraphilic disorders; other mental disorders; medication-induced movement disorders and other adverse effects of medication; and other conditions that may be a focus of clinical attention. You will notice that some of these categories overlap considerably with the domain of neurology. This is unsurprising: with advances in medical technology (especially in fields like molecular biology), the dividing-line between anatomical 'structure' and physiological 'function' is increasingly hard to draw. This is more or less what Charcot expected would happen.

To give you a feel for what a typical psychiatric syndrome looks like nowadays, here are the DSM-5 criteria for major depressive disorder:

The individual must be experiencing five or more symptoms during the same two-week period, and at least one of the symptoms should be either (1) depressed mood or (2) loss of interest or pleasure.

1. Depressed mood most of the day, nearly every day.
2. Markedly diminished interest or pleasure in all, or almost all, activities most of the day, nearly every day.
3. Significant weight loss when not dieting, or weight gain, or decrease or increase in appetite nearly every day.
4. A slowing down of thought and a reduction of physical movement (observable by others, not merely subjective feelings of restlessness or being slowed down).

5. Fatigue or loss of energy nearly every day.
6. Feelings of worthlessness or excessive or inappropriate guilt nearly every day.
7. Diminished ability to think or concentrate, or indecisiveness, nearly every day.
8. Recurrent thoughts of death, recurrent suicidal ideation without a specific plan, or a suicide attempt or a specific plan for committing suicide.

Teddy P, the case described at the start of this book, met these diagnostic criteria. So did Thomas W.

According to Charcot, once we have described and classified such a clinical constellation, and when medical technology has advanced enough to show us the processes occurring inside the brain that are associated with it, we can set about searching for the physiological causes even of disorders like this. Today, we have a plethora of methods for doing so. fMRI and PET, for example, easily allow us to observe in real time the workings of the brain of a depressed versus an autistic or a post-traumatic or a sociopathic or any other kind of psychiatric patient, and see how their neurodynamics, their patterns of activation and neuromodulation, and so on, differ.*

The time would seem to have come, then, to transform psychiatry from an immaterial to a material specialism. What have we found?

The answers are rather disappointing. Modern brain-imaging technology has revealed that people suffering from major depression, for example, show decreased activation of the outer convexity of the cortex and increased activation in deeper brain structures. There is little agreement as to whether this is a *cause* or an *effect* of the illness. If a patient is showing diminished interest in almost

---

* Interestingly, the neurodynamics do tend to be echoed by the brain's haemodynamics.

all activities and experiencing excessive feelings of worthlessness and guilt, discovering that the part of the cortex that deals with the outside world is less active than the part that deals with inner feelings and ruminations is not discovering very much. It's a bit like discovering that the language area of your brain lights up when you are speaking.

A more interesting finding is that, among the deep brain structures just mentioned, an area called the 'subcallosal cingulate cortex' tends to be overactive in people suffering from major depression. This is the closest thing we have found to a 'dynamic lesion' of the kind that Charcot had in mind. Accordingly, a neurologist named Helen Mayberg placed electrodes in the white matter beneath this area of the cortex. Her aim was to artificially decrease activity in the overactive part, and commensurately increase activity in the underactive parts with which the subcallosal cingulate cortex is richly connected.

In her initial experiments she achieved good effects. Subsequent investigators obtained more mixed results, however, and the first major double-blind randomized controlled trial was abandoned after six months, on the basis of a 'futility analysis': only 20% of patients who received the deep brain stimulation (DBS) showed clinical improvement, compared to 17% of those who received sham stimulation, so it was judged unethical to continue the trial.[17]

What this means for Mayberg's theory is anybody's guess. I will point out just two things. First, her initial experiments (in which she achieved a 66% success rate)[18] were conducted on an 'open label' basis – which means that the patients knew they were receiving a treatment for which their doctor had high hopes. (It also means that they had an established *relationship* with her.) The second thing is that Mayberg quickly came to the conclusion, even after her relatively successful initial experiments, that the symptomatic improvement brought about by DBS was only sustainable if it was followed by a course of psychotherapy. As she pointed out to me at the time, such patients are incapable of using psychotherapy at the start of the experiment because they are too under-energized and pessimistic. After stimulation, they are suddenly able to engage in other forms of treatment. Mayberg explained:

> This brings up a critical point about this new treatment. DBS is not a cure-all, despite how robust the clinical responses appear to be. The DBS starts the process by normalizing a very dysfunctional circuit. For full functional recovery, you also need to get adequate rehabilitation, as provided, for instance, by CBT [which is, of course, a form of psychotherapy].[19]

The same applies to ECT and antidepressant medications like SSRIs: they can open a window of opportunity, but they are not a cure.

So much for dynamic lesions. And so much, perhaps, for the dream of making psychiatry a physiological discipline, in which mental diseases can be deduced from brain scans as easily as pregnancies can be read off an ultrasound. But if there is no physiological lesion in the brain, how can we make sense of what these disorders actually are?

A reasonable place to look instead, I believe, starts with a *psychological* observation that is made in the DSM-5 definition of major depressive disorder, just after the diagnostic criteria listed above:

> Although there is a clear distinction to be made between depression and sadness, it is possible for major depressive disorder to occur in addition to sadness *resulting from a significant loss, such as bereavement*, financial ruin, or a serious medical illness. The decision as to whether a diagnosis of depression should be made will depend on the judgment of the clinician treating the individual.[20]

In other words, we *do* know what causes depression, or something very like it. We routinely encounter the same symptoms and signs (depressed mood, diminished interest or pleasure in activities, decreased or increased appetite, a slowing down of thought, a reduction of physical movement and so on) following *a significant loss, such as a bereavement*. It only registers as a disorder when it seems excessive or contextually inappropriate. In fact, since there is nothing to the definition of depression beyond these diagnostic criteria, we might as well boil them down and say that depression is simply *grief* where we can't work out what has been lost. This relationship between depression and grief was even starker in the DSM-4 definition, which stipulated (under 'criterion E') that the diagnosis of major depression should be made only if 'the symptoms are not better accounted for by bereavement, i.e. after the loss of a loved one'.

This might not be the *physiological* cause that some are looking for, but it is surely significant that essentially the same group of feelings, thoughts and behaviours that we call 'major depressive disorder' occurs naturally and normally when we lose a loved one. This suggests that we might profitably re-direct our search for the causal mechanisms of depression toward the functions performed by the brain circuits of attachment, about which we now know quite a lot. The regulation of these circuits cannot be separated from early life experience. We know, for example, without a shadow of doubt, that clinically depressed people have – on average – suffered significantly more 'adverse childhood experiences' (centrally including separation distress) than non-depressed people,[21] and we know that women are more than twice as prone to depression than men (remember: women CARE more, on average). We also know that the first depressive episode is usually triggered by an experience of loss.

You can't pretend that attachment has nothing to do with the psyche. Freud was very struck by the connection between depression and attachment, a connection that the authors of the DSM appear to concede: pathological depression ('melancholia') in its clinical manifestations is strikingly similar to normal grief (to 'mourning').[22] This suggests that the *cause* of depression is no less psychological than physiological.[23] Current mainstream psychiatry elides this fact, and treats depression as though it were caused by a physiological 'disease of the forebrain' – conflating 'function' with 'physiology' – a scientific fudge that just happens to be convenient for the pharmaceutical industry.

Today the most widely accepted theory in psychiatry (and in the general public, by extension) about what causes depression is that it is produced by a 'chemical imbalance'. To be specific, it is said to be caused by a deficiency in the neurochemical *serotonin*.

The idea that functional disorders might be caused by chemical imbalances is entirely consistent with Meynert's vision. Likewise, unbalanced neurotransmitters (the very existence of which was unknown to 19th-century doctors) are precisely the sort of thing that Charcot predicted future doctors would be able to see: dynamic physiological processes during life that do not produce lasting anatomical damage, but which influence the same brain tissues that structural lesions do.

Unfortunately, the reasoning behind the 'serotonin deficiency' hypothesis – first proposed in 1967 and popularised when the selective serotonin re-uptake inhibitor (SSRI) Prozac came to market in the 1980s – is faulty. In its simplest form, it goes like this: since antidepressant drugs like Prozac decrease the symptoms of major depression, and since these drugs increase the level of serotonin in the brain, depression must be caused by a deficiency in serotonin.

Where to start? If a patient's chest hurts when they exert themselves (a syndrome called 'angina pectoris'), a decent cardiologist will not prescribe painkillers. That treatment might bring temporary relief from the symptoms, but eventually the patient will die of the underlying disease. This is because the disease is *caused* by a narrowing of the arteries that supply the heart muscle with blood, preventing it from getting the oxygen it needs. Accordingly, the appropriate treatment is surgery to bypass or expand the narrowed vessels. This operation relieves the pain, and the attendant risk of death by cardiac arrest, by removing its cause. Merely suppressing its symptoms using pain medication – let alone claiming that they are caused by a deficiency of endogenous analgesics – would be medically illiterate and very dangerous.

Generalize from this example, and you see the difference between *symptomatic* and *causal* therapy. Ordinarily, as soon as a symptomatic therapy such as a pain medication is withdrawn, the symptom returns. Once a causal therapy such as bypass surgery or stenting is introduced, by contrast, the symptom is more or less permanently cured. The chemical imbalance hypothesis is therefore logically faulty: it mistakes a symptomatic therapy for a causal one, and then misidentifies the cause.

It has also been discredited empirically. The respected journal *Molecular Psychiatry* recently published an 'umbrella analysis'[24] of all the available evidence, conducted by Joanna Moncrieff, a leading British psychiatrist. It showed that depleting serotonin in normal people does not cause depression. It showed also that depressed and non-depressed people do not differ in terms of anything to do with serotonin: they have the same amounts of it, and of serotonin transporters and receptors, and of the genes that produce these things. She concluded:

> Our view is that patients should not be told that depression is caused by low serotonin or by a chemical imbalance, and they should not be led to believe that antidepressants work by targeting these unproven abnormalities. We do not understand what antidepressants are doing to the brain exactly, and giving people this sort of misinformation prevents them from making an informed decision about whether to take antidepressants or not.[25]

Despite all this, psychiatrists today almost exclusively treat depression and other mental disorders using drugs. In other words, they tinker with your brain chemistry: serotonin in most antidepressant medicines, dopamine in almost all antipsychotic medicines, noradrenaline (known as 'norepinephrine' in America) in many anti-anxiety medicines – and, in tandem with serotonin and dopamine, in some antidepressant and antipsychotic medicines too.

Let's pause for a moment and ask a question with a sceptical ring to it. *Is this so bad?* These are, after all, the same neurochemicals that I have noted already are the currency of our affective circuitry. These circuits produce the bad feelings that we want to avoid, but frustration of the emotional needs they represent won't kill us. In the depths of evolutionary time we might have been at risk from predators and abandonment in the desert wastes; not so much now. If our emotional needs aren't *needs*-needs – actual necessities for survival – why not just take a pill to make the feelings go away?

In the last year of his life, Freud wrote:

> We are concerned with therapy only insofar as it works by psychological means; and for the time being we have no other. The future may teach us to exercise a direct influence, by means of particular chemical substances, on the amounts of energy and their distribution in the mental apparatus. It may be that there are other still undreamt-of possibilities of therapy. But for the moment we have nothing better at our disposal than the technique of psychoanalysis, and for that reason, in spite of its limitations, it should not be despised.[26]

The most obvious sign that psychopharmacological therapy is symptomatic rather than causal is that the symptoms usually return as soon as the drug is withdrawn. That would be fine if they were provoked by a passing crisis, but most common psychiatric disorders are chronic: they go on indefinitely. As a result, it is far from unusual (indeed, it has become normal) for people to take psychoactive drugs for decades.

On the whole, this is not how their application was originally specified. Psychiatrists were therefore not always prepared for the side effects caused by protracted use, such as the terrible movement disorders caused by long-term antipsychotic medication – acknowledged in the DSM-5 with its own class of 'disorder' (disorders caused by the medication).* They also didn't anticipate the significant difficulties that arise when you try to take patients off drugs such as benzodiazepines and SSRIs. Habituation to some classes of psychiatric drugs (for example, many anxiolytics and most hypnotics) means that we must keep increasing the dosage to achieve the same results. And of course, some psychoactive drugs (opiates, for example) are frankly addictive.

This last remark raises an uncomfortable parallel between psychiatric medication and self-medication through drugs of abuse. Drugs like opium and cocaine provide artificial ways of satisfying, respectively, the attachment and exploratory drives. In effect they *mask* the symptoms of separation distress or attention deficit, instead of addressing their causes. There is no fundamental difference between opium and cocaine on the one hand, and, on the other, medical opiates and psychostimulants of the kind that were once liberally recommended for emotional disorders, and which still are prescribed with abandon for ADHD.

I drew attention, just a few pages ago, to the fact that the artificial suppression of feelings like panic and despair by self-administered narcotics is a 'defence' mechanism. So let's put it bluntly. The mainstay of modern psychiatry – psychopharmacology – is for the most part a *defence* against facing the facts about what our patients really need. It is a way of suppressing symptoms instead of asking what they mean and fixing that. And as we saw in Chapter Four, most psychopharmaceuticals are not very effective anyway.

Why, if all this is true, would mainstream practitioners of a whole branch of medicine take such an approach? In my opinion, the answer is twofold. First, many psychiatrists today still believe, as Freud's old teacher Meynert did, that what really ails their patients 'transcends the bounds of accurate scientific investigation'. Second, like Meynert, they still believe that the treatment that their patients really need 'implies more than we can accomplish'.

---

* Consider the case of Teddy P, in this respect.

And yet – as we saw in Chapter Four – we *can* accomplish it, by following essentially the same procedure that Freud developed on the basis of his largely (though not entirely) vindicated inferences about the workings of the mental apparatus.

The most compelling evidence that he was on the right track is of course the 'sleeper effect': patients who have been treated using psychoanalysis tend to *keep getting better*. This is what we would expect from a causal rather than a symptomatic therapy. Bad feelings tell us that there is something about how we are living that doesn't meet our own needs, something that deep habits of mind prevent us from addressing or even perceiving. Like stenting a coronary artery, helping a patient to forge new mental pathways relieves their pain by removing the blockage that is the real culprit.

Perhaps this sounds a bit sweeping. It would of course be absurd to say that there is no place in modern psychiatry for drugs. There are illnesses whose causes are simply unknown: autism* and schizophrenia are paradigmatic examples. The decades-long quest to find a structural basis for either one of them is the career graveyard of neuropathologists. Does this mean that they are ultimately psychodynamic in origin? I think it's only fair to say that the jury is still out. Whatever their causes, however, they often entail cognitive impairments which make it extremely difficult for the patients to formulate flexible and realistic predictions or to participate in the collaborative work that psychotherapy entails. Therefore, for the present at least, symptomatic treatments are essential.

This is a good moment to reflect briefly on whether these diseases are well defined in the first place. Are they even real? Here I think Charcot's approach remains the most promising: careful

---

* I am referring to severe cases of infantile autism, of the kind originally described by Leo Kanner. The term 'autism spectrum disorder' refers to a very wide range of clinical pictures.

description and classification of the symptoms and signs that constitute coherent syndromes. This is the DSM approach. But what renders a syndrome 'coherent' in the rest of medicine is the fact that it reliably indicates the presence of a specific pathological-anatomical process. It is precisely this that is lacking in psychiatry; hence the endless search for 'dynamic' lesions.

Freud's approach, I need hardly remind you, was different. He didn't merely describe and classify the different clinical constellations, he *analysed* them (as did Luria, who called it 'syndrome analysis'). The aim of such psychological analyses is to identify the underlying component functions – the dysfunctions which explain the surface picture. The DSM fails dismally on this front.

Here is one striking example. A common denominator in the syndromes of major depression, panic disorder and OCD is *separation distress** – which suggests that these three clinical entities belong in the same broad class of disorders. The component function that is implicated in these syndromes is the attachment drive, which does have an identifiable physiological correlate. And yet they are classified in three entirely different classes in DSM-5. In my view, given the present state of mental science, the seven basic categories of emotional need are the most fundamental natural kinds upon which we can base our psychiatric categories.

Returning now to schizophrenia and autism: even if they are construed as physiological diseases, this is not to imply that they are accessible *only* to symptomatic treatments, or that environmental factors play *no* causal role in them. For example, if the cause of autism is a congenital cognitive disability – inability to formulate and flexibly update context-sensitive predictions, say – then the feelings that this deficit produces might tend to lead the child to avoid the stress of unpredictable settings, such as social situations, and to narrow their field of engagement to the most predictable ones (computers, perhaps, or train timetables). That would be a *defence*. 'Organic' causes do not preclude a role for psychodynamic

---

* The anxiety in OCD is mainly of the 'panic' rather than the 'fear' variety (see Jackson & Solms, 2013).

mechanisms in the progression of any mental disorder, as we saw even in the example of anosognosia caused by stroke.

Drugs can be useful in many other psychiatric conditions, too. Some patients are so ill that they cannot make use of the causal therapies they need, either because they take too long to be effective (for instance, in cases of acute suicidality) or because they require more active engagement than the patient can muster (as with severe depression). The fact that the functional mechanism of attachment – for example – is both physiological and psychological means that it is possible to treat it both physiologically and psychologically. After seeing the disappointing results from serotonin-boosting drugs, the psychoanalyst and psychiatrist Yoram Yovell – working with Jaak Panksepp – proposed that low doses of a relatively safe opiate called buprenorphine might be an effective drug against suicidality, on the hypothesis that it is an extreme form of 'protest' behaviour. (Recall that the 'protest' phase of the separation-distress response is mediated by mu opioids.) The results were encouraging (effect size = 0.58).[27]

I also don't want to leave you with the impression that *no* psychiatric illnesses originate in a 'chemical imbalance'. We are not all born the same. Just as some of us are born to be short or tall, so too some of us are born more fearful, more aggressive, or more clingy, than others. In other words, some of us are born with more sensitive brain emotion circuits of one kind or another. That doesn't absolve us of our developmental obligation to learn how to meet these emotional needs; it just makes the task more difficult.

Last, I don't mean to suggest that psychopharmacology is the only symptomatic treatment that is used in modern psychiatry. In fact, most treatments in psychiatry are symptomatic: that goes for electroconvulsive therapy and transcranial magnetic stimulation and even for vagus nerve stimulation – and also for some forms of psychotherapy. It includes, for example, the widespread use of purely behavioural approaches in the treatment of addictions, phobias, anorexia nervosa, sexual dysfunction, sleep disorders, PTSD, OCD, social anxiety, and many other emotional disorders.

These behavioural treatments have their place in our therapeutic arsenal. Even though most of the disorders just listed have developmental origins, when the root causes have been addressed we are sometimes still left with symptoms. Disorders can take on a life of their own, as they become complicated by secondary mechanisms. Once you have treated the emotional cause of an addiction, for example, you still must treat the physiological dependency itself. Insomnia might ultimately be caused by separation anxiety, but eventually, secondary worries about not being able to fall asleep start to play a part too. In such cases, when the patients have successfully completed a causal therapy, I sometimes recommend a symptomatic treatment to round things off.

The same applies the other way around. Psychogenic erectile dysfunction, for example, is readily treated with drugs, but purely pharmacological treatment fails to address the deeper emotional factors that caused it in the first place – especially in younger men. These cases require psychotherapy even when the presenting symptom (pipe down) is no longer the major concern. To take an extreme example: imagine what would have happened in the case of Johan T – assuming that the cause of his sexual inhibitions was erectile dysfunction – if he was treated only with Viagra.

The starting point of psychiatry cannot be the study of brain functions, and still less the molecular biology of neurotransmission or neuromodulation. What is distinctive about psychiatry is that, unlike neurology, it treats the *psychological* manifestations of *functional* pathologies of the nervous system. This obliges it to base its treatments on a theoretical understanding of the functions of the psyche.

When Hobson claimed that the causal mechanism of dreams was 'not psychological but physiological'[28] he displayed remarkable conceptual naivety. Think of my dream about the lost letter from my late father (p. 53); how could its cause have been physiological? Of course, it manifested itself in both psychological and physiological events, but it was obviously *caused* by the history of my relationship with my father. When I reported this dream to my analyst, I was overcome by sadness, and I started to sob. That, too, in a sense, was a physiological event. But is the physiology of the tear duct (or the neural mechanisms that control it) the best way to understand what happened? Take the sadness I felt about my dead father, multiply the intensity and duration by a factor of ten, and then you have 'major depression'. Is that best understood physiologically, or would it make more sense to understand it in terms of the psychological mechanisms of attachment, separation and loss? Those mechanisms, as we have seen, are physiological, too, but the functional laws that govern them cannot be reduced to molecular biology.

Psychiatry has always been sensitive about its scientific credentials, precisely because – no matter what Meynert said – its fundamental mission is to treat the soul. Freud tried to provide a framework for accomplishing this mission scientifically, not by replacing the soul with the brain but rather by accepting that the 'soul' – construed as the experiencing, active, living 'I' – is a part of nature. On this basis, he set about studying its internal construction, using a naturalistic method, and drawing theoretical inferences from his observations, just as one does in any other science. This enabled him to construct a model of the mind in terms of its functions: its underlying component parts, the dynamic relations between them, and the forces and energies that drive them.

In doing so, he was following the advice of his revered teacher,[29] the great physiologist Ernst von Brücke, as reported in 1842 by Emil du Bois-Reymond:

> Brücke and I pledged a solemn oath to put into effect this truth: 'No other forces than the common physical and chemical ones are active within the organism. In those cases which cannot currently be explained by these forces one has either to find the specific way or form of their action by means of the physical-mathematical method *or to assume new forces equal in dignity* to the chemical-physical forces inherent in matter, reducible to the forces of attraction and repulsion.'[30]

The great problem of 'falsifiability' that dogged the psychoanalytic model of the mental apparatus and its workings – in health and disease – was a problem with Freud's method, not with his theory. This problem has been overcome by virtue of a singular fact which Freud himself recognized: the apparatus of the mind, and only of the mind, can be studied both from the subjective and from the objective perspective. For this reason, although the subjective perspective was his necessary starting point, Freud looked forward to the day when his theoretical model could be tested, supplemented and corrected by physiological methods of investigation that were not yet available.

The methodological advances that I am talking about now make it possible, in principle, to verify objectively the existence (or not) of 'repressed' ideas, for example. It should be possible to ask a psychoanalyst who has interviewed patients with pathological grief reactions – and who has on this basis inferred the repressed ideas lying behind their symptoms – to provide a list of words which denote those ideas, and then test whether the patients' brains respond to them differently from 'control' words (for example, matched words that refer to their explicit symptoms rather than their implicit causes). An EEG technique called 'evoked response potentials' (ERP) could be used for this purpose. It may be predicted that, if the inferred repressed ideas really do exist, they should evoke different brain responses from the control words. If that does not occur, the existence of the so-called repressed ideas will have been falsified.

I say this should be possible in principle. Well, guess what: it has been done in practice, by a psychoanalyst named Howard Shevrin.[31] What he showed is that not only does the brain respond differently to the inferred repressed ideas, as predicted, it also responds particularly quickly and strongly to them when the words are presented 'subliminally' (that is, *unconsciously*, by means of a tachistoscope, which presents visual stimuli so briefly that the research participants see nothing consciously). The opposite pattern of responses occurs with the control words: the brain ERPs are weaker and slower when these words are presented unconsciously – and stronger and quicker when they are presented consciously.

I said earlier that Freud's peers rejected his notion of 'unconscious ideas' – not only on empirical grounds but also on logical ones. The term was considered to be an oxymoron: an unconscious idea is not an 'idea', it is a set of neuronal connections that becomes an idea only when it (somehow) emerges in consciousness. However, evidence of the kind just cited has led the modern neuroscientific community to fully accept the existence of unconscious ideas. If reading meaningful words, and understanding them, and responding differentially to them, do not qualify as 'mental' functions, then it is hard to say what does.

Psychiatry can't evade the fact that the mind is a mind. Biological psychiatry's attempts to suppress feelings chemically rather than to understand what's causing them and address that, its claims that dreams are random epiphenomena, that the infantile origins of our adult thoughts and behaviours have no bearing on our mental health, and so on, is a remarkable piece of denial – a defence. But against what?

When Freud introduced 'psychical reality' into science, he could only study functional disorders subjectively. His inferences about what lies behind these disorders – what causes them, what explains them – could, in those days, not be tested objectively. He had no objective methods for studying the functional dynamics of the living brain. Rather than speculate about the underlying dynamics in physiological terms, as Meynert did, or wait forever, as Charcot did, Freud felt obliged on both conceptual and empirical grounds to study them from the subjective perspective. But this was not meant to be the end of the matter. I have quoted this passage (or parts of it) before:

> We need not feel greatly disturbed in judging our speculation upon the life and death drives by the fact that so many bewildering and obscure processes occur in it [. . .] This is merely due to our being obliged to operate with the scientific terms, that is to say with the figurative language, peculiar

to psychology (or, more precisely, to depth psychology). We could not otherwise describe the processes in question at all, and indeed we could not even become aware of them. The deficiencies in our description would probably vanish if we were already in a position to replace the psychological terms by physiological and chemical ones.[32]

Elsewhere, he wrote: 'We must recollect that all of our provisional ideas in psychology will presumably one day be based on an organic substructure.'[33]

Sadly, this is not how subsequent generations of his scientific followers saw it. They believed that his aim was to develop a purely psychological psychiatry, when in fact he did so only *provisionally*, awaiting the development of physiological methods that were equal to the problem. This is not because Freud believed that the brain is *more real* than the mind, but rather because it is easier to study objectively.

So it happened that 'biological' psychiatry and psychoanalysis developed along parallel tracks, with neither side wanting anything to do with the other. When neuroscience finally developed the physiological tools needed to test Freud's ideas, his followers took no notice. Their failure to engage with these advances left Meynert's scientific heirs to their own devices, not to use these miraculous instruments to find the long-sought missing links* between our subjective and objective perspectives on the actual causes of mental illnesses, but rather to double down on the idea that 'you' – your mind – does not *really* exist. Ever since, its main business has been the development and promotion of pharmacological products to suppress every sign of suffering, with unsurprisingly troubling results.

And psychoanalysis? By then, it was on a frolic of its own.

---

* Freud once wrote to Georg Groddeck: 'The unconscious is the long-sought missing link between the physical and the mental' (letter dated June 5, 1917).

CHAPTER SEVEN
The Future of an Illusion

PATIENT: How shall I live now? I've lost my life-concept completely. I don't understand how this could happen. I was ready for any blow. You have no idea how much I've had to work to achieve everything. I never had anything for free. Previously, I had a particular value system. I used to know exactly what is good and what is bad, what is wrong and what is right, what is acceptable and what is unacceptable. Nowadays, if someone describes some life situation to me, it's no longer clear to me what attitude I should adopt toward it.
— *From the author's clinical files*

Lord N was a retired captain of industry, in his eighties by the time I saw him. He had achieved a great deal in his long life, won many honours, and should have been enjoying a peaceful retirement. Instead, he kept waking in the night, disturbed by a thief in his house.

His wife thought it was a recurring dream that he was mistaking for reality. His doctor wanted me to assess him for a sleep disorder. Just going by the description, though, the problem sounded more serious than that. The old man had taken to getting out of bed, stomping around his large house and garden, searching for this intruder, whom he had come to believe was a young boy. He bawled out his security guards: 'What the hell is the point of employing you if you can't keep that little shit away?' It was getting embarrassing. The family feared a scandal.

When I examined him, I found many signs of cognitive

impairment and many more of paranoia. Alongside his nocturnal episodes, he kept calling for meetings with his accountants and lawyers, demanding proof that his funds were not being misappropriated, that his properties had not been sold off. He said he knew that his former right hand – the CEO of a public company for which Lord N had served as chairman – had sold out to a rival firm. He knew this, he said, because he had seen it on television. But he couldn't have done, for no such event had taken place and no such report was broadcast. The confusions descended mainly at night and in the early evenings, a phenomenon called 'sundowning'.

Considering his multiple vascular risk factors and the clinical neuropsychological picture, I suspected vascular dementia. An MRI confirmed my hunch: multiple small blood vessels had ruptured deep within the white matter and basal ganglia of his brain. Confusional episodes, mainly at night, are part and parcel of the syndrome, especially the type that is caused by small-vessel disease. The tissue damage was irreversible, but we wanted to impede further decline by managing the underlying vascular pathology. To this end, Lord N stoically consented to various medications and a strict diet. All the same, the thought of that spectral boy running around the estate at night nagged at me. Something psychodynamic must be going on, too. I recommended a parallel course of psychotherapy.

Lord N saw me weekly. He was guarded at first, but soon came to speak quite freely about his many suspicions. We covered, of course, the story of his life, and I did my best to conceal my impatience for clues to the nature of his intruder. Did this scoundrel bring anyone particular to mind, I asked? 'Toynbee perhaps,' he said after a long pause. 'Robert Toynbee.' This turned out to be a boy he remembered from boarding school. 'Why does he remind you of Toynbee?' I asked. 'No idea,' he said.

As the session proceeded, we quickly got on to the subject of Lord N's children, in particular his eldest. This young man had proved something of a disappointment. It wasn't that he lacked ambition; if anything, his manoeuvrings on the board of Lord N's former company had shown a little too much of it. He had recently had the temerity to suggest that his father should transfer all his remaining shares to him, to facilitate a takeover. 'He's behaving as if I'm dead already,' said Lord N. His daughters, too, had openly haggled in his presence about who was going to get which favourite property.

I suggested that the 'intruder' might stand for his son, or perhaps for his children in general. 'You might have a point. That boy can be quite shameless.' After a moment's reflection, he added: 'I have just remembered something about Toynbee. I was the school squash champion until that little shit usurped me!'

All these impatient young usurpers. The underlying theme was clear: *something is being taken from me*. It didn't seem too hard to work out what, but I wondered whether he was capable of looking directly at it. Lord N was an intimidating man; I was wary about pushing him. All the same, I didn't feel that I could offer him any mere bromides. It was clear that he wanted the truth, as I saw it.

Within a few sessions I felt bold enough to observe that he was indeed being robbed of something, by the deterioration of his brain. 'It's natural that you should feel anxious,' I said. 'You're losing your grip, and you're no longer completely sure what's going on.' To my relief, he agreed, and seemed reassured by my candour. At the very least, this solved for him the mystery of why he was so powerless to stop the intruder. Encouraged, I went on. 'It's not only your intellectual grasp that's going. You've also lost your position. You're no longer the one who calls the shots. It must be difficult to adjust to that; to your reduced place in the world. It might feel humiliating, perhaps even enraging.' Again, he agreed that this was how it was.

In a subsequent session I explained how, at night, when we are sleeping or have just woken up, the brain doesn't fire on all cylinders. Top-down 'executive' control goes away almost entirely during sleep, which is why our worst fears – the worries that we suppress during the day – pop up so vividly in our dreams. 'That's why you have those nocturnal visits from the burglar. Your worry about losing your grip comes to the fore while you're sleeping, and then, when you wake up, you can't think your way out of it, as you would have done when you were in better command of your faculties.' Lord N was persuaded. 'So, there really isn't a burglar. I *see* him instead of *thinking* about what's really on my mind.' 'That's it exactly,' I replied.

In the sessions that followed, a deeper anxiety surfaced. It wasn't only his authority that he was losing; it was his grip on life itself. Few things can be more terrifying. Lord N wasn't afflicted by the extreme death anxiety that dogged my youth, but he was now facing the truth that, no matter how omnipotent he had once been, he wasn't long for this world. After talking about this topic for several sessions, we agreed to call it a day.

The whole treatment lasted only a few months. Brief as it was, though, I consider it a remarkable success. It wasn't that the disturbances at night had ceased; they hadn't. Yet, now when Lord N woke up, he was able to tell himself that the intruder was just an illusion, conjured by his mind to concretize his more diffuse worries. He could address himself to those in the light of morning. Then he would turn over and go back to sleep. The anxiety and confusional symptoms had largely melted away, even if the vultures were still circling.

It's ironic that, despite all the attention he gave to the subject of figures of fatherly authority, Freud struggled to come up with a workable succession plan for his own intellectual estates. Many remarkably eccentric schools of psychoanalysis have arisen over the years, all claiming descent from him, if not exclusive rights to his legacy. True to the pattern of an Oedipus complex handled badly, they were mainly either slavish in their loyalty or chaotically rebellious and subversive. In some cases, they were both. Freud wondered whether this wasn't inevitable: 'You have only to think of the strong emotional factors that make it hard for many people to fit themselves in with others or to subordinate themselves.'[1]

The first and best known of the rival schools developed from

Freud's split with Carl Jung. Jung was a gifted young researcher at the Burghölzli hospital in Zurich, under Eugen Bleuler, then one of the world's leading psychiatrists. Freud saw Jung as his ideal heir, not only because he was a psychiatrist (most of his other pupils were neurologists) but also because Jung was a Christian and therefore a useful rebuttal to the antisemitic claim that psychoanalysis was 'Jewish science'.

After collaborating closely for several years (1907–13), during which time Freud secured Jung's appointment as president of the newly formed International Psychoanalytical Association (IPA), the two men parted ways. Freud accused Jung of denying the importance of infantile sexuality, and worse, of mysticism. Jung accused Freud of pathologizing unconscious mental processes, and worse, of dogmatism. (There were many other mutual charges but these were the main ones.) After their break, Jung founded the school of 'analytical psychology', which is associated with such concepts as the collective unconscious, universal archetypes, synchronicity, and the extrovert/introvert distinction.

The last of these was adopted as one of the axes in the popular Myers-Briggs personality quiz, which sounds less mystical than some of Jung's other ideas, though in fact it is rooted in the four elements of ancient cosmology. If he ever learned of it, Jung probably would have enjoyed this association. Not for nothing is he called the 'founding father of the New Age'. He reported near-death experiences, participated in séances, collaborated with ESP (extra-sensory perception) researchers and believed in poltergeists. He also developed a theoretical system to explain paranormal occurrences and incorporated astrology into his therapeutic work. He wrote:

> By mapping out the positions of the planets and their relations to one another, together with the distribution of the signs of the zodiac at the cardinal points, [the birth chart] gives a picture first of the psychic and then of the physical constitution of the individual.[2]

His interest in Gnosticism* was so strong that the Jung Foundation purchased a Gnostic scroll – one of the 4th-century Nag Hammadi volumes that were illegally exported from Egypt – and named it the 'Jung Codex'. (It was returned in the end.)

Despite the rather strange views that Jung ended up espousing, my own reading of his falling out with Freud is that – at least initially – it had more to do with personal rivalry than anything of scientific substance. Freud ended up tacitly agreeing with his challenger's early view that the sexual and self-preservative drives were basically indistinguishable and, like Jung, he ultimately found that most unconscious processes were well adapted to their tasks.

Perhaps the compatibility of the later Freud with the earlier Jung partly explains why, despite my 'Freudian' credentials, I am often invited to speak at Jungian conferences. The audiences tend to receive my neuroscientific findings concerning dreams, drives, the unconscious and more with respect and positive interest, and (slightly to my regret) I have never witnessed anything overtly thaumaturgical. Even their dress sense is disappointingly similar to that of the Freudians: no greater preponderance of floaty garments or headscarves.

Following Jung's departure, a string of other rival schools similarly arose from fallings-out between Freud and his more ambitious pupils. Alfred Adler created a diagnostic framework in which everything comes down to inferiority complexes. Wilhelm Stekel built one that was all about unconscious symbolism. For Otto Rank, the trauma of birth was the main thing. On the whole, these schools did not endure, though Adler's name has seen a revival in popular interest thanks to the bestselling Japanese self-help book *The Courage to be Disliked*.[3] Wilhelm Reich could also be grouped with these early dissidents – it's all about 'orgone' energy – but he developed his esoteric views and broke with the psychoanalytic mainstream only after Freud's death.

---

* Gnosticism is a religious and philosophical movement that emerged in the 1st and 2nd centuries CE; it is characterized by an emphasis on personal spiritual knowledge versus institutionalized religion.

Who, then, was Freud's 'true' successor? Probably his daughter, Anna. During and after World War II, she worked with war orphans in London, co-founding the Hampstead War Nurseries and later the Hampstead Child Therapy Course and Clinic (now the Anna Freud Centre). Here, she developed methods for observing and treating children based on such orthodox Freudian premises as the importance of developmental stages, the role of the environment, and the adaptive capacity of the ego. Freud might have been a little surprised that it was Anna who ended up as the de facto boss of psychoanalysis. Her scientific contributions during his lifetime were not very substantial, and her later authority probably derived more from her surname – and her unwavering loyalty to him – than from any original contributions of her own.

The same cannot be said of Melanie Klein, who was the first of Freud's pupils to develop a genuinely significant rival school of child psychoanalysis. One of her many detractors in the Freud circle described her as 'a Polish housewife with fantasies'.[4] In fact, she was born in Vienna (in 1882), and it was her family's financial difficulties that pushed her into early marriage and motherhood, depriving her of a medical education. This no doubt put her in a precarious position among the would-be heirs to the Freudian legacy.

Klein never challenged Sigmund's authority directly; in fact she went to great lengths to argue that she was more Freudian than Anna was.[5] The compliment was not reciprocated. In the ugly theoretical and technical disputes that erupted between Klein and his daughter, Freud unequivocally sided with Anna. His principal objection to Klein was that her speculations about the mental life of pre-verbal children could never be verified. As he insisted, the very fact that these children were pre-verbal meant that they were in no position to confirm or correct anything she said about them.

Kleinian psychoanalysts comprised the majority of my teachers in London. How they came to so dominate the British Psychoanalytical Society is anybody's guess, but I can confirm from personal experience that they are frightfully *certain* of their views; not only on theoretical matters, but even in the interpretations they make to their patients. These can be quite alarming. Traditional Kleinians place an extraordinary emphasis on the destructive side of human nature, even in tiny babies, in whom they postulate something called 'primary envy'. According to them, babies think that the mother's breast cruelly keeps most of its goodness and richness for itself, and consequently they are mad with fury much of the time. Daniel Stern, an eminent researcher of early mental development based in Switzerland, once observed that it was remarkable how differently babies in London thought from those in Geneva.

In the many clinical presentations that I attended during my 14 years in London, I was struck by how often my Kleinian colleagues conceptualized their cases as *the patient envying the analyst*.* Whenever I queried the evidence for these pervasive conclusions – very tentatively, as a candidate – it invariably met a retort to the effect that I wasn't *really* an analyst. I never knew whether this was because I was a neuroscientist, a candidate, or a candidate whose analyst was so closely aligned with Anna Freud that it placed me beyond redemption.

Whatever the truth, it seems to me that there really is a challenge to the scientific aspirations of psychoanalysis in this very assertive style of inference. If we insist on our own judgement too strongly, we will struggle to see past our ideas to the true complexity of the situations before us. (Is this baby tormented by envy, or wind?) At the same time, there is clearly a balance to be struck. On the same grounds that Freud criticized Klein, my neuroscience colleagues sometimes insist that we can never be sure what animals feel, or indeed whether they feel anything. How could we ever know the mental states of non-verbal beings?

Here I tend to side with the Kleinians, who note that the same applies to the interpretation of anything that is unconscious – or, for that matter, anything that is unspoken. In ordinary life, we assume that we have *some* ability to judge the emotions and thoughts of others from nonverbal evidence. I think there is an interesting,

---

* For the patient's perspective (or at least *one* patient's perspective) see Michael Bacon's (2024) harrowing account of his analysis.

not-to-be-taken-for-granted respect in which we really can see through the attitudes of a face or body to something of the inner world. It doesn't work all the time, and of course deliberate deception (such as pretending) is possible. Yet the possibility of deception presumably implies a default relationship that is reliable. Very young children tend to be extraordinarily demonstrative, pantomiming their emotions with startling clarity. A standard part of psychoanalytic training is simply to observe a baby once a week over the course of the first 12 months of life. The point, of course, is to learn what's underneath all our encrustations of adult conditioning. I wonder what effect such training might have on neuroscientists who deny the existence of basic emotions. At any rate, if psychologists deny evidential value regarding subjective states to anything except verbal reports, we are on a slippery slope back to behaviourism, and perhaps to a debilitating credulity in everyday life.

How to resolve this dilemma? Trick question, it isn't one. We can in fact consider more than one kind of information. Obviously, in search of converging lines of evidence, we must test our hypotheses using *multiple* research methods, each one offsetting the weaknesses of the others. We would need good reasons to reject any seemingly relevant observations from decent research. So, we must accept that nonverbal evidence is genuine evidence about internal states, albeit with difficulties that we should take into account when we weigh it.

By the light of this principle of heterodoxy, it's a shame that, on the one occasion that Melanie Klein and Anna Freud ever agreed on a point of theoretical importance, they ended up on the wrong side of the question. In the 1950s, a young psychoanalyst named John Bowlby (later an *eminence grise* in the biological field of ethology) argued that babies and mothers have an innate *drive to attach*, independent of the sexual drive and the drive to feed.*
Klein and Anna Freud both objected to this idea: it was clear to them that Bowlby had to be wrong, because (said Anna) he was

---

* Bowlby was here following in the footsteps of an older British analyst named Ronald Fairbairn.

contradicting Sigmund Freud's conclusion that babies take pleasure in feeding only because it is libidinized, through 'anaclisis', and the same must apply to tactile and visual contact with the mother as well.

Bowlby had in fact provided overwhelming behavioural and experimental evidence that falsified Sigmund Freud's view, not only from direct observation of human babies and children, but also of other primates.* You might think this would have settled the matter; but alas, the point upon which Melanie Klein and Anna Freud were firmly united was precisely that Bowlby's evidence was inadmissible, having been obtained by non-psychoanalytic methods. Just because babies (and monkeys) are distressed by *actual* separation from their mothers, Klein argued, doesn't mean that the distress is caused by the separation itself; it might equally be caused by *fantasies* the baby has about the absent mother (which in her view were plausibly that the baby's envious hatred had driven her away).

From the standpoint of science, this is obviously a shoddy position. What is puzzling is that it was also bad as dogmatic orthodoxy. Sigmund Freud made numerous statements to the effect that the drives could not be classified on the basis of psychological data alone, since their taxonomy was fundamentally a biological question. In 1915, for instance, he wrote:

> I am altogether doubtful whether any decisive pointers for the differentiation and classification of the drives can be arrived at on the basis of working over the psychological material. This working over seems rather itself to call for the application to the material of definite assumptions concerning the life of the drives, and it would be a desirable thing if those assumptions could be taken from some other branch of knowledge and carried over to psychology.[6]

---

* See Bowlby & Robertson's film *A Two-Year-Old Goes to Hospital* (1952), a painful illustration of how hospitalized children were treated at the time – as I can confirm from my own experience at the age of two.

If Melanie Klein and Anna Freud wanted to defend the classical purity of their doctrine, why not that part? Regardless, later neuroscientific research demonstrated that Bowlby was right and that Freud and Klein were wrong. Bowlby is now cherished as one of psychoanalysis's great pioneers, and the Freud/Klein consensus has been conveniently forgotten. I can imagine worse outcomes.

The Kleinians invite criticism for dismissing verbal reports too lightly, putting too much trust in clinical intuition (construed as 'countertransference'). But what happens when an analyst takes words too seriously? What if each utterance were submitted to an immense crushing weight of interpretation?

In 1963, the IPA took the drastic step of expelling the French psychiatrist Jacques Lacan, formally stripping him of the right to call himself a psychoanalyst. Its main complaint was his innovation of 'variable length' consultations. At Lacan's whim these might end at any moment; a tactic, so he claimed, to break his patients out of their habitual defences. Behind this procedural irregularity, however, lay a wilderness of theoretical deviations, at the centre of which lay the question of the place of language in mental life.

Born in Paris in 1901, Lacan came to psychoanalysis via psychiatry and a distinctively Left-Bank assortment of cultural influences: Surrealist art, Symbolist poetry, and the philosophies of Hegel and Heidegger. For both of these proto-existentialist thinkers, the distinction between mind and world breaks down in unsettling ways. Simplifying a little, Hegel said that the world was nothing more than the universal mind coming to recognize itself, and Heidegger said it wasn't even that: mind and world both melted into a 'fundamental ontology' of appearances. This must have been heady stuff for a young doctor trained in physiological psychiatry. Yet there was a final ingredient that might tip any excitable character over the edge: Lacan also got very interested in the linguistic theories of Ferdinand de Saussure.

Saussure had argued that the meaning of an individual expression was determined by the relationship between the parts of that expression and the parts of every other possible one. That is, it was determined by the abstract structure of the language. *Meaning*, on this account, depends on *structure*. And what is the mind if not structure? Come to that, what is the world if not structure? What *couldn't* structure be?

Such was the baggage that Lacan brought to psychoanalysis. In his famous theoretical seminars in Paris, attended by the brightest and coolest, he reinterpreted psychoanalytic theory, focusing on Freud's texts in a way that calls to mind the cabalistic spirals of schizophrenia. Freud, for instance, once wrote that *Wo Es war soll Ich werden* (in the canonical translation, 'Where id was, there ego shall be'; or 'Where *it* was, there *I* shall be' if you're Bruno Bettelheim).[7] This slogan has usually been interpreted as meaning that the goal of analysis is to replace the troublesome impulses of the id and the automatic responses of the unconscious mind with conscious decisions. To clarify the point, Freud remarked that the process was 'not unlike the draining of the Zuider Zee', drawing a then-topical analogy with the Dutch government's reclamation of dry land from a shallow inlet of the North Sea.

Passing in silence over the obvious, Lacan suggested several alternative translations for these six words. In particular, he pressed the questions of why Freud had not used the eight-word alternative *Wo das Es war soll das Ich werden* ('Where *the* id was, there *the* ego shall be'), and why *werden* had been translated as 'be' rather than 'become'. Surely the omission of the articles was important, Lacan insisted. Why else would Freud have capitalized *Es* and *Ich*, thus indicating that these words were not to be read as pronouns (since, in German, one capitalizes ordinary nouns but not pronouns)? He elaborated:

> The true meaning would seem to be the following: *Wo* (Where) *Es* (the subject—devoid of any *das* or other objectivating article) *war* (was—it is a locus of being that is referred to here, and that in this locus) *soll* (must—that is, a duty in the moral sense,

as is confirmed by the single sentence that follows and brings the chapter to a close) *Ich* (I, there must I—just as one declared, 'this am I,' before saying, 'it is I') *werden* (become—that is to say, not occur (*survenir*), or even happen (*advenir*), but emerge (*venir au jour*) from this very locus in so far as it is a locus of being).[8]

Finally, Lacan rendered his own gloss on this unexpectedly slippery remark: 'Being of non-being, that is how *I* as subject comes on the scene, conjugated with the double aporia of a true survival that is abolished by knowledge of itself, and by a discourse in which it is death that sustains existence.'[9]

Reading this, you might have the slight feeling of being led up a dark alley the more discreetly to mug you, but Lacan never seems to have suffered a moment's doubt in this patter-physics. Indeed, it was clear to him that the more usual way of interpreting Freud's aphorism was itself an Anglo-American plot.*

Many people took Lacan very seriously. Many still do; I would hazard a guess that there are at least as many Lacanian psychoanalysts in the world today as there are any other brand. It is easy to recognize a classic Lacanian: they almost always wear black, and they speak in the gnomic style of the master. Some of them, like my old professor Jean-Pierre de la Porte, add a French accent.

Is there anything to all this? Because Lacan is so hard to read, it's hard to be sure. Yet there probably are some nutritious morsels hiding in his Zuider salad. I have suggested that one of Freud's most important lessons to neuroscience is that unconscious thoughts can usefully be considered as *thoughts*, not just physiological states. What would it mean to see them that way? Lacan's famous answer is that 'the unconscious is structured like a language': that is, its associations are riddled with puns and codes, its patterns are like the patterns in texts, and so on. This must be true, at least to some degree. I doubt what Lacan believed, namely that the unconscious consists in little more than language-like

---

* Recall the definition of paranoia in Chapter Five.

structures all the way down. For one thing, we ought to expect that it contains lots of structures that are more like dance steps, given its central role in automatized action. Yet the question of *how much* of it is like language, and which parts, and in what ways: these are fine topics for research.

So, arguably, is Lacan's contention that experience comes to us filtered through the prisms of our semantic categories, and that these in turn gain meaning from the entire symbolic architecture of our cultures. The question of how far 'observation is theory-laden', to use a perfidiously Anglo-American statement of this idea, was a major theme of late 20th-century psychology and philosophy of science. It led to interesting scientific work on everything from unconscious racial bias to the categorization of gender. Yet less attention has been paid to the thing that most interested Lacan: the point where the cloud of symbols parts for a moment, and something from *outside* interrupts our habits of mind. What happens when words fail us? What happens when we encounter 'The Real'?

It is in the context of all this that we must consider the unsettling character of Lacan's actual treatments. The verbal nitpicking wasn't confined to the written texts of theoretical forebears: words uttered in analysis were routinely battered senseless, too. As if that weren't bad enough, Lacan was known to physically strike some of his patients. According to a former student, he once literally kicked a woman out of his consulting room. Then there are those 'variable length' sessions. Towards the end of his career, another student relates, they might last just five minutes, Lacan hovering in the doorway throughout. The analyst and author Jacques-Alain Miller said that '[Lacan]'s morality derives from a superior cynicism.'[10] A charitable assessment might well see him in the dog-bites-dullard tradition of Diogenes the Cynic, whose outrages were meant to shock ancient Athenians out of the habitual absurdities of custom. We might also think of him as a kind of Zen practitioner, whose non-sequiturs startle wisdom-seekers out of the prison of conditioned thought and thence to enlightenment. Then again, perhaps he was just a bully.

If 'superior cynicism' is what you want, that might be reason enough to involve yourself with Lacan's legacy. There are others. Parts of it are profound. Parts are obnoxious, and seem to license a cryptic obnoxiousness in adherents, which they might even enjoy. There's a Nouvelle Vague aesthetic to the whole thing, and an Oulipo trickiness. My requirements as a psychoanalyst are more humdrum. At the risk of betraying a naive concern with the *hors-texte*, as Lacan's heir Jacques Derrida liked to call reality, I want to know: does this stuff work? Is a person suffering from mental illness going to get better if they go to a therapist from this anti-school school? On theoretical grounds, there is reason to imagine they might. The resemblance to the lessons of ancient sages hints at some sort of wisdom. Lacan's departures from the Freudian script could turn out to be helpful, even if we would hesitate to call some of them ethical.

The trouble is, we don't know. This approach to therapy is highly individualized, which makes it hard to design meaningful studies. Vanishingly little research has been done, and few Lacanian practitioners seem interested in changing that. When the IPA turfed Lacan out in 1963, they were in effect safeguarding their own *appellation contrôlée*. I'm inclined to think it was the right call. Who could meaningfully vouch for such a rogue element? Consider this a label warning: if it isn't from a certified analyst, it's just sparkling bite-whine. *Cave lacanem.*

Still other schools emerged, though unlike those of the earlier charismatic theorists, they no longer seemed to emanate from Oedipal revolts. In many cases it was now quite easy to guess what lay behind the language: applications for new funding, pitches for new markets. The most recent one, which came to prominence in the 1990s, is called the 'relational' school. As far as I can tell, it is barely distinguishable from the object-relations, interpersonal and intersubjective schools, dating respectively from the 1920s, 1930s and 1980s. This latest approach is said to represent a 'paradigm shift'[11] away from classical psychoanalysis because it 'assigns primary importance to real interpersonal relations, rather than to instinctual drives'.[12]

Two significant claims are embedded in this bland-sounding statement. The first is that drives are not 'real' – at least not in the sense that interpersonal relations apparently are. The second is that the basic elements of experience are literally constituted through these interpersonal relations.

Relational analysts emphasize that theirs is a 'two person' psychology, by contrast with the 'one person' model of classical psychoanalysis. On this view, whereas classical analysts see the drives and affects as originating *within* the person, relational analysts conceptualize them as originating developmentally *between* people. You can see the essence of the idea in a commonplace scenario. If a child trips and grazes her knee, she looks towards her carer to determine what this means. If the carer looks alarmed and hugs her, the child infers that grazed knees are painful enough to elicit sympathy; if they merely raise an eyebrow and put her back on her feet, she absorbs the lesson that they are no big deal and that one just gets on with life.

Classical psychoanalysis has a complicated quasi-mechanical model to explain this difference. In the first situation, the child learns to associate the perception of having taken a tumble and the experience of pain with the relief of being comforted and attended to. That association heightens the salience of pain-feelings after falls, turning them into opportunities to satisfy a desire. The child focuses on the pain and makes a fuss, not out of cunning or duplicity, but because the whole unconscious sequence of actions works *because* it hurts. In the second situation, the child finds that there's nothing to be gained by dwelling on small upsets, and so the pain of the graze can't hold her attention. She must learn other ways to obtain the pleasure of attention, or the relief of getting out of rough-and-tumble games.

What a lot of invisible machinery! Isn't it simpler just to say, like the relational school, that the experience of the pain is actually created by attention from the carer, and that we learn to feel whatever our caregivers seem to expect? On further thought, however, this move has some far-reaching, rather weird corollaries. If subjective qualities as apparently basic as pain are not given naturally, but instead are 'constructed' within early relationships, what reality do any of these feelings have? What are they constructed out of? Desires and anxieties and everything else that constitutes the life of the mind become mere shadows of the intersubjective contexts in which they developed.*

Relational analysts believe that we re-create (or 'enact') these early contexts in our subsequent adult lives. For this reason, they focus on helping their patients to become aware of these enactments in order to break out of troublesome patterns. So far so good; I doubt whether any psychoanalyst would claim a different goal. Where the relational school stands apart is that its analysts would never try to infer the historical *facts* of a patient's development, let alone make generalizations about the objective workings of the mental apparatus. Rather, they seek 'mutual construction of meaning in the analytic relationship'.[13] The analytic investigation of transference is – in their view – no less intersubjectively co-constructed than the original childhood events were.

This is the crux of the matter. Where Freud sought to *include* 'psychical reality' in our objective picture of the human organism, some staunch relational psychoanalysts seem to assume that *everything* is psychical: that there is no such thing as an objective reality when it comes to the life of the mind. No fact of the matter about what you felt, why you acted as you did, or indeed what happened next. No structure anywhere! A fog fills the head. If there are no determinate facts about the mind, nothing can be determinately associated with material states of the brain. Then again, perhaps the brain *has* no such states – how could one know, except by looking at a scan or an autopsy? Yet surely *seeing* is also an intersubjectively co-constructed experience, with no more credible a connection to reality than anything else. The fog escapes the skull and fills the universe – if there even is such a

---

* Lisa Feldman Barrett, you might recall, takes a similar view.

thing. One begins to sympathize with Meynert, the behaviourists, and every other bid to exorcize the mental sciences of such vast, billowing spirits.

Do the practitioners of the relational approach worry about these implications of their theory? Who knows. Even to ask the question seems to contradict their basic premise – or perhaps it depends who's asking. Most of them, in my experience, are simply trying to be nice to their patients, to be modest about what they 'know', to recognize that we are all in the same boat and none of us is captain. In short, my guess is that the main aim of relational psychoanalysts is to set themselves apart from the stereotype of bullying, arrogant, know-it-all doctors of the mind.

If that's all it is – a policy of not saying much about reality, in the interests of intellectual humility, or a marketable facsimile thereof – I'm happy to leave them to it. Still, if it *is* just an attempt to differentiate their style of therapy from the bad old days, it's puzzling branding. The basic approach certainly isn't new. Even the foggy philosophy rings a bell. If, in a weak moment, we try to take it too seriously, we find ourselves on a not-so-royal road that we have taken several times already.

Why do the tribes of psychoanalysis keep getting lost among the shades and shapes of a dream world? It's not just the relational school. The classic Lacanians strongly resemble an occult sect, poring over their arcane writings, burrowing away to reach an unimaginable other side of the other side. Jung embraced the paranormal with both arms. Even the Kleinians have a gnostic streak, especially those who follow the teachings of Wilfred Bion, who correctly observed that we can never know reality in itself and that scientific investigation therefore involves an 'act of faith', but whose hardcore acolytes may seem to believe that he (and perhaps only he) really did know the final truth.

It could be argued that Freud invited this esoteric tendency. He was the one who taught us that experience is full of mysterious messages, meant for us yet often eluding our grasp. There is of course a sense in which any Freudian account of the mind must give a certain 'idealist' temperament its due. The world *as we experience it* surely is a construction of our minds. Be that as it may, Freud unequivocally wanted psychoanalysis to be a science, by which I mean a sincere attempt to get to grips with the reality that generates experience.

That aim was, I think, the right one. There's no guarantee that we will ever get to the ultimate answers about what's real and how things work. Reality might not be set up in such a way that we could; it would be bad luck, in a certain sense, but it's imaginable. (We have been imagining such bad luck at least since Descartes declared that there was only one inference he could be sure of: that he thought, therefore he was.) All the same, the task of scientific knowledge, rather like that of life itself, is to avoid serious error. Let our mistakes be cheap and illuminating! And if we must have faith in something, we could do worse than putting it in ourselves.

When it comes to the science of the mind, having faith in ourselves means trusting that we can work out the nature of our position and respond accordingly. Faith in anything else means relinquishing agency.* It abandons the aspiration to use our intelligence to work out where we stand – both our individual situation in life, and the place of the mind in the rest of nature. There may be comfort in doing that, or relief, or liberation of a kind. It may even be healthy, in certain situations. But if we stop testing our ideas against the world, grow indifferent to the accuracy of our predictions, the achievability of our wishes, the evidence of our senses, then I think we have, in a sad and dangerous way, given up. We live by getting life right enough to live. It takes effort; we can't rest easy with ideas that are wrong, or not even wrong. Unchecked delusion is a crack in the engine block of our selves: soon enough, the unforeseen will come rushing in.

Saying this, I can't help noticing the resemblance between

---

* Freud saw belief in God as a transference of our infantile faith in omniscient, omnipotent and infinitely beneficent parents.

Popper's concept of falsifiability and Freud's 'reality-testing'. It makes sense, though: what is science, but the institutional form of our obligation to accommodate things as they are, which Freud called the reality principle? As he observed, in a slightly different context:

> We welcome illusions because they spare us unpleasurable feelings, and enable us to enjoy satisfactions instead. We must not complain, then, if now and again they come into collision with some portion of reality, and are shattered against it.[14]

In light of all this, let's turn at last to a loose end that has been trailing for a couple of chapters now. Freud thought that the root of every mental disturbance was frustrated sexual desire. He was flat wrong, I think, about the nature and number of our drives. This is another way of saying that he *didn't know what we need*. The necessities of life were not only what he thought they were. In which case, how on earth did the talking cure ever work? And why does it demonstrably work now, even when implemented by psychoanalysts who remain in thrall to his outdated conjectures?

It doesn't always go well, of course. It's certainly possible to do bad therapy. We can make our patients worse-off, through misfortune, incompetence, or by abusing the power and authority of our position. The stakes are as high as they are in any other form of psychiatric care. And yet, for all this, there is always an odd sense that, while what we do in psychoanalysis matters very much, objective *reality* is not so important.

That's a cryptic remark. An example should make the point clearer.

Suppose you are consulted by a patient whose fear circuit is pathologically active, putting them in a constant state of anxiety. What would be the best way to cure them? There are two commonsensical 'objective' options. The first is to use drugs to disable the circuit or block its signals. This is what benzodiazepines do:

they objectively target the part of the brain that causes fear. It works well, for as long as the drugs are active. Yet the anxiety tends to return as soon as the patient comes off them (as would be wise, given their side effects and risk of addiction). Also, as the chronicle of SM's misadventures with Urbach–Wiethe disease suggests, it's useful to have a capacity for fear. Fear has a job to do. Life is hard when you can't feel the risk of risky situations. Whatever it is, then, the pharmacological approach clearly isn't a genuine cure.

The second 'objective' option is that you can try to make the patient really, really safe. The fear circuit exists to make us avoid danger. Once we give it what it wants, it should stop complaining. Isn't that logical? Yet somehow this doesn't work, either. In fact the whole problem with a patient suffering from an anxiety disorder such as PTSD is that they are afraid even when they are already safe. I once had a patient who went to inordinate lengths almost every day to ensure that he was safe from mortar fire, a decade after he was last on any battlefield. What is it that patients like him need?

What they need is to *feel* safe. That requires something subtler than literal safety, but it also requires something less dishonest (as it were) than switching off the part of the brain that allows them to feel afraid. To make them feel safe in a lasting, well-adjusted way, we need to help them alter the system of ideas (perhaps deeply consolidated and unconscious) that mean *for them* that they are always in danger. This is their predictive model. How exactly it implies this omnipresent threat will be a product of many factors that are personal to the patient, ranging in scope from memories of instructive experiences to the whole philosophical atmosphere of their mind, ending perhaps in their metaphysical beliefs. Not everyone in the battalion who survived the mortars emerged, as my patient did, with PTSD; the way in which he personally experienced this bombardment turned out to have much to do with his earlier life experiences.

Here we come face to face with the strange detachment of mental life from the objective state of things. It is neither feasible nor desirable to 'correct' a patient's entire outlook, to bring it into line with the analyst's personal take on reality. In that sense, the views of the individual analyst matter far less than those of the patient. One can try, at most, to carve a few new paths through the forest of predictions that lie between the patient's feelings and the outside world they are living in now. A judicious firebreak here and there and we might free someone a little from the formative events of their past. Yet even that much change can take immense effort. There's no option to erase the whole thing and start again. The analyst can only work with what they find.

Having worked a good deal on the drives, I sometimes get a bee in my bonnet about how useful it is to know what they are drives *to*, and I often wish psychoanalysts paid more attention to developments in neuroscience generally.* But the cure is never simply to give the drive what it wants. On the contrary, we try to reveal to the patient their own systems of ideas, so that they can recognize and accept the ideas as theirs, and rethink them where necessary, until their experience of reality can pass *their* tests, and give them what they need, per the definitions in *their* predictive model: their idea of safety, their idea of a good time, their idea of love, and so on. I grudgingly accept that the theoretical grounding an analyst needs to do this probably doesn't include a deep grasp of the workings of the brain, any more than you need to know how a microchip works to change someone's computer system settings.

In this sense, the skill of doing analysis is less like science and more like a practical trade. Long experience leads to familiarity with many different kinds of glitch and suggests many different kinds of fix. Working in one culture or community will teach

---

* For example, all the drives – as we understand them in affective neuroscience today – are relational. 'Object relations' are implicit in them: the FEAR drive implies a threatening object; the RAGE drive implies a frustrating object; the PANIC/GRIEF drive implies a caregiving object; etc. The individualized way in which we learn to satisfy these drives is therefore intrinsically object-related. The dichotomy between 'one person' and 'two person' psychologies thereby loses its premise.

analysts a lot about how that community thinks, and how to work with such thoughts. The lessons might not travel, but they would still be very useful in the right clinical context.

Some problems can also reveal quite general things about the underlying functioning of the brain. Look how much Freud was able to work out simply by talking to his patients and listening carefully. I suspect that psychoanalysis still has a lot to contribute to brain research, which is why I hope that at least some practising analysts keep abreast of the questions that preoccupy other mental scientists. But it may be that psychoanalysis always had more to teach neuroscience than the other way around.

It may even turn out that, through careful attention to what happens at the neurophysiological level during moments of breakthrough and processes of transformation, we could at last learn how to cure mental illnesses by acting directly on the brain. What if we could isolate what an effective talking cure does to your pathways and gradients, and then manipulate the grey matter to replicate that effect? Towards the end of his life, Freud seemed quite optimistic about this prospect. We have already seen what he wrote in 1938:

> We are concerned with therapy only insofar as it works by psychological means; and for the time being we have no other. The future may teach us to exercise a direct influence, by means of particular chemical substances, on the amounts of energy and their distribution in the mental apparatus. It may be that there are other still undreamt-of possibilities of therapy. But for the moment we have nothing better at our disposal than the technique of psychoanalysis, and for that reason, in spite of its limitations, it should not be despised.[15]

I hope I have persuaded you to be cautious about betting against Freud, but here I think there are grounds to doubt his vision. One lesson that psychoanalysis teaches again and again is that experience itself matters. Even in our dreams, we try to bind every possible source of free energy arising from the daily disparities between what we believe and what we experience. The inconsistencies tend to have their revenge.

In any case, we're a long way from the day when neuroscience can dispense with psychoanalysis 'at last' and take charge of our souls single-handedly.

I have my own place, of course, among the tribes of psychoanalysis. In one sense I am a fairly direct intellectual descendant of Freud: we followed a similar professional trajectory, from basic neuroscience through clinical neurology and neuropsychology to psychoanalysis. I suppose I could be seen as a Freudian fundamentalist, seeking to return my erring brethren to the true meaning of his texts. And yet I am also part of a less easily defined consortium of analysts and neuroscientists who are persuaded that we can work together productively. In fact, this is what I have spent much of the last four decades doing, under the banner of 'neuropsychoanalysis'.

When I completed my early research on the brain mechanisms of sleep and dreaming, and undertook clinical training in psychoanalysis, I had no one to talk to except for my then-wife, Karen Kaplan, a junior neuropsychologist like me, who was undergoing training in child analysis at the Anna Freud Centre in London. I quickly learnt that it was unwise to talk to my psychoanalytic teachers about neuroscience. So, after reading the neurologist Oliver Sacks's (1984) book *A Leg to Stand On*, in which he spoke of neuropsychology ignoring the psyche, I wrote him a letter, and we hit it off.

I wrote also to Mortimer Ostow, mentioned previously, an analyst who had undertaken research in the 1950s into the implications of the psychopharmacological treatments that were then just beginning to take root in psychiatry. He invited me to present my dream research findings at the New York Academy of Medicine. In the audience was Arnold Pfeffer, a neuropsychiatrist who (like Ostow) had trained in psychoanalysis in the late 1940s. Pfeffer invited me to address a small group of like-minded colleagues, who gathered monthly at the New York Psychoanalytic Institute to discuss neuroscientific topics relevant to psychoanalysis, under the leadership of James Schwartz, co-editor of Eric Kandel's monumental textbook *Principles of Neural Science*.

This was in the early 1990s. In a series of lectures to this group, over the ensuing months, I reported findings arising from the psychoanalyses of personality changes in patients with variously-located brain lesions. Soon, I was convening the New York group in Schwartz's stead. (This is how I came to enjoy those monthly meetings with Kurt Eissler.)

Ostow knew Kandel personally, which is how I learnt of Kandel's opinion that 'psychoanalysis still represents the most coherent and intellectually satisfying view of the mind'. This was a few years before he won the Nobel Prize, in 2000, and before he published his recommendation that psychiatry in the 21st century should be based on an integration of psychoanalysis and neuroscience. Our monthly meetings – which involved an increasingly wide circle of psychoanalysts, neurologists and neuroscientists, including Jaak Panksepp – began to attract international interest.

In 1999 we set up a journal, edited by Edward Nersessian and me, with the title *Neuropsychoanalysis* (the first time the word was used). That led to the establishment of an International Neuropsychoanalysis Society, which held its first congress at the Royal College of Surgeons of England. The keynote speakers at the first congress were Oliver Sacks, Jaak Panksepp, Antonio Damasio and Clifford Yorke, plus me. They all joined the advisory board of the journal, along with many other luminaries such as Kandel, Ramachandran and LeDoux on the neuroscientific side, and Charles Brenner, André Green and Peter Fonagy on the psychoanalytic side. (Just about all the other researchers I have mentioned in this book did likewise, including Karl Friston, Mortimer Ostow, Helen Mayberg, Howard Shevrin and Yoram Yovell.) At the time of writing, the International Neuropsychoanalysis Society, in its 26th year, has 1,138 active members.

What unites us is the conviction that it is time to return to the huge task that Freud abandoned over a century ago, owing to the lack of suitable empirical methods. How do the details of Freud's functional model of the mind match up with our deepening knowledge of the physiological, chemical, genetic and epigenetic workings of the brain? As you have seen throughout this book, we use multiple research methods to explore the neurophysiology of psychodynamic processes, and the psychodynamics of neurophysiological processes. We scan the dreaming brain, we psychoanalyse patients with focal neurological lesions, we measure the electrophysiological signatures of repressed conflicts, we manipulate the chemistries that mediate our basic emotional drives, we vary our psychotherapeutic techniques in line with advances in understanding of how the brain changes, then measure the results, and so on.

On this basis, can we now write the chapters that were omitted from Luria's great textbook? I sometimes wonder why any of my psychoanalytic and neuropsychological colleagues bother to do anything else. The scientific discoveries and clinical insights arising from our ongoing interdisciplinary work are too numerous to summarize here. I have mentioned some of the breakthroughs, such as the wishful mechanism of dreams and of confabulatory amnesia, the defensive aspect of anosognosia, the role of separation distress in the brain mechanisms of depression (and in addiction, panic disorder and OCD) and its implications for psychopharmacology, the physical (informational) nature of the 'functional' mechanism in functional neurological disorders, the empirical verification of repression, the developmental neurobiology of infantile amnesia, some neural constituents of empathy, the deep connections between drive and consciousness, not to mention a tentative solution of the 'hard problem' of consciousness. Some other puzzles are works in progress – such as our currently ongoing research into the neurophysiology of free association, the biological function of dreaming and the possibility of artificial consciousness.

Most gratifying is the fact that psychoanalytic therapy for

neurological and neurosurgical patients is becoming increasingly commonplace, as I can only hope it will once again for psychiatric patients. It is also good to see the growing number of psychoanalysts and psychotherapists – from all schools – who have adjusted their techniques to accommodate our insights into the therapeutic action of the talking cure. In my own career as a working therapist, I have found that some of my most interesting and rewarding cases were ones in which it really mattered exactly where and how brain meets mind.

About a year after my sessions with Lord N finished, I ran into his wife at a public event and asked how he was. Nowadays, she said, the worst that happened when he woke up was that he put on his lamp to read. 'He's not the man I fell in love with,' she said. 'But honestly, his thinking in general has really improved. He's much less confused about everything.'

This shouldn't have surprised me as much as it did: psychotherapy can't reverse cognitive decline, but cognitive deficits can be greatly exacerbated by emotional distress. Even so, the idea that mere conversation could have helped my patient to this degree struck me as a sort of magic. A rare feeling: power.

After a moment's silence, Lady N said, 'He has also been having some conversations with me about our mortality.' I asked what these conversations had been about. She looked uneasy, then came out with it. '*No matter how much you might have achieved in life,*' she said, '*no matter who you are. In the end, it comes to this.* That's what he told me.' A wincing sort of smile, both of us. What can you say to that? We clasped hands and bade each other farewell, and let the movement of the party sweep us off to our different lives.

'The end' is a question of perspective. Lord N died more than a decade ago. I never spoke to him again, yet he has often been in my thoughts – for his public triumphs much more than our brief alliance.

We care about our legacies precisely because they go on after us. What should we live for, knowing that, in the end, it comes to this? What should we leave behind us?

As it happens, Freud has some useful lessons here, too.

CHAPTER EIGHT
A Cure by Love

PATIENT: We've had several incidents in the last week where I had to run away from my little girl into another room. She bit me yesterday. It was so interesting. It was like I could feel something rush through my body. I felt – I don't know how to describe it. Almost 'dulcet'? I was completely off, but I also felt so calm. It was bizarre. I felt like that for the rest of the day.
ANALYST: Did you notice any other emotion in yourself?
PATIENT: I don't know how to describe it. I wasn't happy, but I felt, in a way, sparkly or something. That's why at first I didn't realize what was going on. Sometimes, I just feel like I'm going to scream at her and I'm going to lose it. It was getting to that point yesterday. I could see that she was ramping up. I could absolutely see it, and I was starting to get angry. Then she looked me straight in the eye. I remember that moment, saying: 'Come here, darling,' and she walked right over to me and bit me. And then it was: 'OK, that's where we are.'
ANALYST: There was a lot of anger in you leading up to that moment, but it seems it was transformed somehow.
PATIENT: It just went away.

— *From the author's clinical files*

Before the First World War, a large chunk of eastern Germany and central Europe consisted of a patchwork of semi-autonomous 'state countries' ruled by Bohemian princes ('Bohemian' in the geographic rather than the evaluative sense). One of these princes, reigning (after the war) over a portion of what was once Lower

Lusatia, situated on the wooded and sparsely peopled North European Plain of the Holy Roman Empire, was named Friedrich III of Solms-Baruth. He was descended from a long line of counts and princes who had ruled the state of Baruth for the previous 300 years, and other Holy Roman states for about 500 years before that.*

His accession in 1920 made Friedrich one of the great landowners of Germany. He possessed 17,300 hectares, including four castles (one of them, his favourite, in Silesia), a steel works, a porcelain factory, a huge dairy, sprawling commercial forests, farmland, ten villages' worth of 'subjects' and an internationally renowned stud.

Friedrich was tall and gaunt. Raised in the Humanist tradition by his father Friedrich II, a close confidant of Kaiser Wilhelm II, he entered the Imperial cavalry as a captain. It was the senseless waste of the First World War that converted him to pacifism. He resigned his commission and became deeply religious, throwing himself into various pet projects in Baruth and Klitschdorf.

Insulated by his wealth and title, Friedrich had reason to feel relatively immune from Hitler's rise. From the start, he was vocal in his disdain. Although steeped in the traditions of the ancient order, a staunch monarchist even after the monarchy was abolished in 1918, he abhorred nationalism. I suspect that his visceral dislike of Hitler was also motivated by classism; he commented frequently about the boorish vulgarity of the Nazi rabble. He barred his employees from joining the NSDAP and prohibited the use of its infamous salute on any of his estates. In 1933, he refused to fly its flag on his castles, and kept refusing even when it was required by law.

At the start of the Second World War in 1939, Friderich forbade the German military from conducting manoeuvres on his lands. When timber and resin were required for the war effort, he

---

* The original family seats, including that of my own branch, were located further west, in the country of Solms, now part of the modern German state of Hesse. So, Friedrich was not ethnically Bohemian; he was of Frankish descent.

refused to supply it. In 1942, he discovered that Russian prisoners of war had been shot in one of his forests, which bordered an internment camp. He was furious, telling the district leader of the party that the Geneva convention must be upheld at all times and that he would personally see to its being respected on his own properties. Soon afterwards, he was accused of 'trying to form a state within the state'. (This was, in a sense, true, because the old feudal states had long since lost their semi-autonomy.) In 1943, the Nazis charged him with sabotaging the war effort, and appointed administrators to take over the running of some of his establishments. Still, he continued to defy them, and he was frequently hauled before the Gestapo for questioning.

Friedrich was not alone among the nobility for his disrespect of Hitler. As the tide of the war turned against Germany, an increasing sense of urgency developed within this elite circle, many of whom were high-ranking officers in the armed forces. (This was conventional in every European aristocracy, which made Friedrich's resignation of his commission all the more unusual.) One of these rebels – not a nobleman – had been a fellow officer with Friedrich during the First World War, where he was shaped by the same terrible experiences. His name was Admiral Wilhelm Canaris, and he was now head of German military intelligence.

Canaris had been secretly undermining Hitler's progress ever since the invasion of Poland in 1939. Now, however, it was clear that more urgent action was called for. Canaris realized that Friedrich's public dissidence provided perfect double deception: the Nazis would never imagine that a group plotting to assassinate Hitler and stage a military coup would be stationed in the house of a known anti-Nazi. So, Friedrich's castle in Baruth, about 70km from Berlin and just 15km from military headquarters, became the plotters' den. Cover for their clandestine meetings and protection from the very real risk of eavesdropping was provided by Friedrich's stud: the plotting by these equestrian aristocrats was conducted on horseback, as they went riding together through Friedrich's forested estate. To further burnish the subterfuge,

Friedrich had his children join the rides, although at a safe 'four horse lengths' behind the adults so they wouldn't overhear their discussions.

In addition to Canaris and others, the conspirators included Erwin Witzleben, Ludwig Beck, Georg Hansen, Carl-Hans Hardenberg, Friedrich-Werner Schulenburg, Henning Tresckow and Claus Stauffenberg, the last of whom actually planted the bomb in the Wolf's Lair near Berlin. The name of Adam Trott should also be remembered, although he does not seem to have been part of the group that met at Baruth. As is well known, Hitler survived the blast, suffering only tattered trousers and a ruptured eardrum. Most of the conspirators – including Trott – were hanged by piano wire or forced to shoot themselves.

The day after the blast, July 21, 1944, the Gestapo came to Baruth to arrest the prince. There were just six of them; they evidently weren't expecting trouble. As two of the officers led Friedrich to where they had parked in front of the castle, his son (nicknamed Fritz, since his official name, too, was Friedrich) was watching from an upstairs window, ready with a hunting rifle. He was a medical student at the time. His father looked up at the window and shook his head, then quietly got into the car. Fritz wasn't sure what the gesture meant. He didn't shoot.

Perhaps that was just as well. Unlike most of his comrades and thousands of others (approximately 7,000 people were arrested in the aftermath of the assassination attempt, and almost 5,000 were executed), Friedrich's life was spared. This was for two reasons. The first was that his wife, Adelheid Schleswig-Holstein, was closely related to the Swedish royal family. Sweden was at that time brokering a secret deal with the chief of the SS to end the war. A message was sent to Heinrich Himmler to the effect that if anything should happen to Friedrich, the consequences for the negotiations 'could not be predicted'. The second reason was that Himmler had an eye on Friedrich's properties. A condition of his release, therefore – after nine months of incarceration and torture in the notorious Prinz Albrechtstrasse prison, and later another prison in Potsdam – was that he had to sign a declaration forfeiting all his properties to the SS, placing them under Himmler's personal control.

On this basis, Friedrich was allowed to leave Germany for Sweden, en route to South Africa, where he eventually settled.[1] Actually, 'settled' is not the right word. Within 18 months he was dead. According to Fritz, the cause of death was survivor's guilt. The more prosaic reason was prostate cancer, for which Friedrich refused treatment.

Today, the Prinz Albrechtstrasse prison has been converted into a museum to the Nazi resistance. In the courtyard, on a plaque in front of a modest statue, the following words appear in German:

> You do not bear the shame.
> You fought back.
> You gave the great,
> forever tireless
> sign of reversion,
> sacrificing your glowing life
> for freedom,
> justice and honour.*

Shame is a social emotion, closely bound up with what Freud called the 'ego ideal'. Like pride, it arises from the comparisons we make between how we wish to be thought of and how we think we actually are (even if only by ourselves). Many authors have sought to distinguish shame from guilt, claiming, for example, that the latter concerns a specific action that one is ashamed of, whereas in the former the sense of perceived badness encompasses one's whole self. To be ashamed, according to this view, is to be ashamed of what you are, not just what you did or failed to do. I'm not convinced that ordinary usage preserves any such distinction: the phrase 'ashamed of what you did' might trigger bad memories but it doesn't sound like bad English. In any case, at the level of

---

* Attributed to Gertrud Kolmar, a German poet who died at Auschwitz in 1943.

affective circuitry, it seems likely that both emotions involve a mixture of perceived social standing, grief, and inwardly directed rage.

And yet, as I have been insisting for some time now, the purpose of emotions is to drive you to meet your needs. The idea of an emotional need that requires you to *die*, whether in the heat of action or later, from shame or survivor's guilt, seems like a profound failure of the theory, even a contradiction in terms. How can we understand such feelings? What biological need could possibly require your own death? And what does our stubborn, sometimes even shameful drive to live amount to?

Friedrich's sacrifice loomed over our family. My relationship with his son Fritz only really got going when we became near neighbours after I returned to South Africa in 2001. I was glad to not be him; what big shoes to fill. *'Your father tried to kill Hitler – what have you done lately?'*

Still, Friedrich almost certainly believed that his soul would live on somewhere else after the death of his body. Whether or not he was right, we can imagine how such a belief might have motivated him to do what he did.

In practice it can be very hard to tell the difference between brain death, coma, the vegetative state and the minimally conscious state. Apart from patients with locked-in syndrome, I don't look after such borderland cases directly, but it's impossible not to be aware of their presence on our ward. The nurses who look after them move more quietly on those shifts, performing their standard checks and ablutions with a visible effort of memory, as if performing an unfamiliar ritual. When you can't be sure if anyone is actually inside the body you're caring for, it takes a kind of faith to keep going.

If I were to tell you that you will fall into a deep coma tomorrow and never come out of it, but that a life-support machine will keep your vital functions ticking over for many years to come, that last part probably won't provide much comfort. When it comes down to it, the mortality of our bodies isn't really what bothers us. What are we, if not our experience of our own being? The important thing, surely, is the mortality of our minds.

This was no doubt the basis of the belief (the wish, the prediction), widespread throughout human history, that our souls might persist indefinitely. Our bodies clearly don't do that, as we can see whenever we encounter the remains of others. I have had more dealings with cadavers than I care to remember, and can confirm that a tendency to disintegrate accounts for a significant portion of their horror. Yet the very subjectivity of inner experience, the precise thing that defends it so formidably against empirical investigation, provides apparent grounds for a sneaky hope. Unlike our mortal bodies, the only soul we can ever really know is our own. Who, then, is to say what becomes of souls in general when the body fails? Might they not, as it were, *go on*?

This asymmetry – the publicness of the body versus the privacy of inner experience – in turn might explain why we tend to identify more with our minds than with our bodies. The solitary confinement of our inner world offers a paradoxical escape hatch from the actuarial certainties of the outer one. To the extent that we want to live forever, we will draw comfort from suggestions that the inner and outer realms are only distantly and tenuously related,* and be troubled by indications that they go hand in glove. We will resist the thought. We will defend ourselves against it. Over the past century, a current in loosely Freud-informed psychology beginning with Ernest Becker (1973) has argued that the most basic features of all human cultures came about precisely for the purpose of blotting out the fear of death, often by quelling the suspicion that it is really the end. As grand accounts of civilization go, this doesn't seem like such an outlandish possibility, and it has never to my knowledge been convincingly refuted. Be that as it may, people don't seem to like working on 'Terror Management

---

* Take the telling euphemism 'gone to another place' and its associated spatial ideas of crossing over, departing, returning home and so on, common in very many cultures.

Theory' very much, no doubt for reasons that the theory itself predicts, and so the programme has rather ground to a halt.

Death is very difficult. Freud called his own discovery that our minds are not transparent to us 'a third blow to humanity's narcissism', after Copernicus's discovery that the earth is not the centre of the universe and Darwin's that humans are not fundamentally distinct from other animals. The idea that our conscious minds are ruled by our unconscious ones is bad enough. How much more of a blow is it if the unconscious starts to look like the mortal body, discovery after discovery pinning our inmost selves to the mortuary slab? I wonder whether something along these lines could account for how psychiatry and psychoanalysis have drifted apart over the years: the former to the brain viewed without a mind, the latter to the mind imagined without a brain. The more we are forced to contemplate the squishy, twitching interstices between grey-matter ganglia and the psyche's shimmering lights, the more mortal we feel. Take this famous assertion by Sir Francis Crick, the co-discoverer of DNA:

> You, your joys and your sorrows, your memories and your ambitions, your sense of personal identity and free will, are in fact no more than the behaviour of a vast assembly of nerve cells and their associated molecules.[2]

He called this The Astonishing Hypothesis, but even I can see that it is in fact a horrible thought, and (notwithstanding the philosophical distinction between materialism and dual-aspect monism) I'm basically on his side. Like Crick, I would have to say that the subjective self is not plausibly free enough of the objective brain to survive its destruction. Sorry. Any project of reuniting the subjective and objective approaches to mental science, however well-founded, will therefore have to reckon with a serious problem: at some level, we would rather not think about this.

(My cardiologist told me recently that I am living in 'extra time'. Given my age, and the fact that I have the same genetic condition that killed my father when he was a good deal younger than I am now, it is likely that most readers of this book will outlive me. Perhaps you already have.)

Freud attracted an impressive array of contradictory accusations: of pseudoscience and overweening scientism, dualism and materialism, social heights and biological depths, taking claims of abuse too seriously and not seriously enough. This isn't in itself reason to conclude that he must be about right, like news organizations who insist that because all sides seem equally dissatisfied they should be praised for their balance. But I do believe it points to something interesting. His legacy evidently renders him somehow both irritating and elusive, both too much and too little.

This may be why, over the years, the question of his overall moral influence has been such a sore point. Recall the titles of some of the books about him – *Why Freud Was Wrong: Sin, Science and Psychoanalysis*, or *Freud: Darkness in the Midst of Vision*. He has been charged with nihilism, replacing religion with a selfish 'therapy culture', and attacking the very fabric of society. No doubt his frank interest in sexual life gave him a louche reputation in some quarters. It's also true that he saw religion as a response to psychological needs rather than supernatural realities, which would tend to undermine more orthodox faiths. His own explanation of the will to live was stark: we want to continue existing because we love our own being, he said, because we are *in love* with ourselves. Our wish for immortality is *narcissism*. I suppose that is quite a shocking view, even now.

Yet any impression one may form of wilfully corrosive, corrupting wildness is a poor match for the historical Freud. When André Breton travelled to Vienna in 1921, hoping to enlist Freud's support for the Surrealist movement, the author was put out to find 'an old man without elegance' in his 'shabby office worthy of the neighbourhood GP'.[3] In short, he found a bourgeois and conventional man of science, with little interest in the artistic provocations that his ideas had inspired. Salvador Dalí met Freud in London in 1938 and was similarly disappointed, reporting that he had almost nothing to say. For his part, Freud commented: 'I have never seen a more complete example of a Spaniard. What a fanatic!' Of his view on Surrealism more generally, he wrote to Stefan Zweig: 'Absolute (let us say 95%, like alcohol) cranks'.[4]

Generations of political radicals have found Freud a vexing ally, too. One can see why they might approach with eagerness. If psychoanalysis gives us a general model of *individual* subjectivity, the question naturally arises of what it might imply for the possibilities of social life on grander scales. Thus, for example, Herbert Marcuse extended the concept of repression to denounce the conformism of life in capitalist societies. Frantz Fanon used psychoanalytic ideas to illuminate the experience of racism. Thinkers as dissimilar as Judith Butler, Slavoj Žižek and Deleuze & Guattari have seen revolutionary potential in the energies that Freud taught us to recognize. And yet, the historical Freud offers scarcely more encouragement to such efforts than he did to his dismayed Surrealist visitors. Many radical minds have been driven to lament, like Deleuze & Guattari, that 'It is as if Freud had drawn back from this world of wild production and explosive desire, wanting at all costs to restore a little order'.[5]

To the extent that Freud had a general view on politics, it was remarkably pessimistic. He didn't like Hitler or Stalin and he said so when it mattered, but he didn't seem to approve of any other political currents very much either. Whether fascist, nationalist, socialist or religious, he considered mass psychology in general 'impulsive, changeable and irritable [. . .] led almost exclusively by the unconscious.'[6] On his gloomy assessment, the public is essentially hypnotized by charismatic leaders, projecting its own narcissistic ego ideals onto them. We idealize our heroes, installing them as surrogates for the perfection that we desire for our own beloved selves. For Freud, this binding force is what defines social formations of almost any kind: 'A primary group [. . .] is a number of individuals who have put one and the same object in place of their ego ideal and have consequently identified themselves with one another.'⁷

If the behaviour of the masses in general amounts to nothing more than this semi-willing enslavement, the prospects for any kind of politics look dim. Freud therefore recommends disidentification with the group. But how can there be politics without groups? And what could be worth dying for, if not a cause larger than oneself? Is this not a counsel of despair?

For my sins, I am currently translating Freud's correspondence with Oskar Pfister, a Swiss pastor. In a letter written to him on October 9, 1918, shortly after the end of the First World War, Freud wrote the following:

> I grant you; ethics are remote from me, and you are a pastor. I do not break my head very much about good and evil, but I have found little that is 'good' about humanity in cross section. In my experience, most people are trash, no matter whether they publicly subscribe to this or that ethical doctrine or to none at all. That is something that you cannot say publicly, or perhaps even think, though your experiences of life can hardly have been different from mine.

At this point you may be wondering whether Freud had anything useful to say about how to live with one another. You might even doubt whether it's worth living with Freud. Granting, for the sake of argument, that his insights are profound, they could still be toxic, even dangerous. If dwelling upon them tends to lower the spirits and dissolve the bonds of fellowship ('most people are trash'!), perhaps they are best reserved for some class of specialists, who can mine them for the common benefit while sparing us the details. Some truths might be better left unknown.

Perhaps uniquely among our planet's inhabitants, humans can reflect upon our motivations. We can, as it were, step outside them and consider them from an abstract point of view. We might, for example, avoid a dangerous situation because we can *think* things like, 'If I were to enter the lion's den, I would probably die, and that is a bad thing, because I love my own existence.' That is unlikely to be our only reason. Presumably we will have the same motivation as just about any other mammal, namely the feeling of fear. Other animals may have little idea why they feel it; they just feel and respond accordingly. But we can ask ourselves what we are doing, and whether we should be doing it, all things considered.

It is possible to get rather lost in our thoughts, however. Even in ancient times, philosophers doubted whether there could be any objective basis for our values, any ultimate difference between good and bad. Just because we feel that something is good, is it *really*? The question seems unanswerable – until we learn to see our subjective worlds as a true part of nature. To a biologist of the mind, such questions look like basic errors.

We now understand that an objective (indeed a famously pitiless) process called evolution shaped all our feelings to serve its own, somewhat tautological ends. We live in order to live. This means that a single value system underwrites all of life: it is bad to die, and good to survive and reproduce.

The way in which feelings underwrite survival suggests that their function is to enable *choice*: to tell us how well or badly any course of action is going for us, and on this basis to change it. This applies to all creatures that are endowed with feeling. Consciously reflecting upon why we feel fear, or anything else, is what the neuroscientist Antonio Damasio calls an 'extended' form of consciousness: it's an add-on, a special custom feature for the human edition. Feeling is the foundation.

Creatures that lack feelings avoid dangerous situations too, but they do so like automata, without any choice in the matter. There is no consensus as to where, exactly, we should draw the line between minded and mindless creatures. Almost all neuroscientists agree that primates are conscious. Most agree that all mammals are. Many agree that all vertebrates are, meaning that even fishes are conscious. Vertebrates (of which mammals are a subset, and of which primates are a further subset) share the same crucial brain anatomy that appears to be what makes you and me conscious: periaqueductal grey, superior colliculi and midbrain locomotor region – collectively known as the 'midbrain decision triangle'.[8] Stimulating and lesioning these structures in other vertebrates has the same behavioural consequences as it has in us.

Beyond vertebrates, however, things get tricky, because invertebrate nervous systems don't possess obvious homologues of this crucial circuitry. Perhaps they have other ways of feeling their ways through life's problems and making their choices. If choice-making (that is, voluntary behaviour) is the criterion by which we should draw the line, then some cephalopods, some insects, some spiders, and some other surprisingly simple creatures would make the cut, too.*

However, there are degrees of freedom. Human beings appear to be *more* conscious than other animals. This is what enables people like the biblical Daniel to endure the lion's den, despite the feeling of fear. Something similar no doubt kicked in for the July 1944 plotters: to know the danger, to feel the fear, and overrule it in favour of other considerations. To enter the Wolf's Lair, even knowing what they knew.

This is what is at stake in Freud's plea that we should include psychical reality in our scientific conception of the universe. On this view, consciousness *does* something; it is the inmost chamber from which, in moments of uncertainty, our decisions emerge. It is ironic that, although Freud is best known for discovering the unconscious, the whole point of psychoanalysis, both as a treatment and as a philosophy of life, was to help us become *more conscious* of what would otherwise operate in the dark: to counteract the

---

* Similar considerations apply to classifying *living* versus *non-living* organisms. Viruses, for example, are generally considered to be not alive, but the fact that this surprises most people reveals that the decision is by no means clear-cut.

mechanisms of defence, and of repression, and of automatism in general. The purpose, as Goethe demanded on his deathbed, is 'More light!'

Central among the automatisms that we must fight is what Freud (mistakenly) called the death drive. Towards the end of his career he came to think that, when life first came into existence, it must have been opposed by an equal and opposite force, a more general backwards tendency: to 'return to the former state of things', also expressed in what he called the 'compulsion to repeat'. This is how he put it:

> It would be in contradiction to the conservative nature of the drives if the goal of life were a state of things which had never yet been attained. On the contrary, it must be an *old* state of things, an initial state from which the living entity has at one time or other departed and to which it is striving to return by the circuitous paths along which its development leads. If we are to take it as a truth that knows no exception that everything living dies for *internal* reasons – becomes inorganic once again – then we shall be compelled to say that *'the aim of all life is death'* and, looking backwards, that *'inanimate things existed before living ones'*.[9]

Physicists grasp the underlying truth that Freud was reaching for in the Second Law of Thermodynamics: that everything tends ultimately to disorder. Our bodies too: from dust to dust. Biologists today also recognize the existence of what is called 'apoptosis': the fact that encoded within the DNA of almost every cell of our bodies is its own preprogrammed death. Even so, it's quite a leap to call this a *drive*, considering the generally accepted definition of 'drive': they are meant to be active forces, demands made upon the mind for work. They strive for one thing only: to maintain us within the bounds of biological viability, to survive and reproduce. The job of our drives is to take care of us. Death can take care of death.

I hope I am being clear: this is not an appeal for enhanced

THE ONLY CURE

narcissism. It is an appeal for greater recognition of the fact that we are not only objects but subjects, too, and for greater appreciation of its profound implications. Consciousness is, as Freud put it, 'a fact without parallel'. It arises only in conditions of uncertainty. In a sense, its opposite – certainty – *is* death. If we knew in advance how to survive in all situations, there would be no need for drives, for uncertainty, or for consciousness. There would be no need for *us*.

Here, then, we find a permanent silver lining to any cloud that might appear on our horizon. Trouble is what summons us into conscious being. Although I have not been able to identify the exact occasion on which Freud uttered the words, he is often quoted as saying: 'One day, in retrospect, the years of struggle will strike you as the most beautiful.' Whether or not he did say this, some such idea is very deeply embedded in his theories. In Freudian analysis, it is when we can bear to be least sure of ourselves that we are most ourselves.

The first mention of a Solms appears in the Lorsch Codex. It records a donation by Rudolfi of Sulmissa to the Catholic church, in the year 788, of a substantial portion of land and associated buildings. That's a long history of landowning. As I write, Prince Friedrich's oldest grandson, my cousin Nickel (also a nickname, since he too was christened Friedrich), is appealing a German administrative court's decision not to return his family's properties following the reunification of Germany. The court found that Nickel's grandfather had legally transferred the properties to his captors and torturers in February 1945, and so there was nothing to be done: an impressively 'German' decision. At the time of writing, appeals have been going on for almost three decades. Without taking a view on the merits of the case, it's hard not to feel that this is a slightly pitiful coda to Friederich's story of courage and sacrifice. Then again, land is complicated, and legacies are even more so.

Seven generations ago, long before the Holy Roman duchies were unified to form modern Germany, my ancestor Johann Adam Solms relocated with his brood from Rhine-Hesse to the Cape Colony, as South Africa was then called. True to the family trade, he and his four sons took farms, and when I say they 'took' them, you might have an inkling what that involved. My ancestors landed in Cape Town itself but then rapidly migrated eastwards, into the lush Overberg region (meaning 'beyond the mountains'). Along the way, they gained several large properties. Some of these were generously granted by the colonial governor, assembly required; others were purchased from existing landowners.

In 2001, after my father's death, I returned from England to South Africa. In so doing, I became the – given my family history, surprisingly unprepared – custodian of a vineyard approximately an hour's drive from Cape Town.[10] While I was growing up in Namibia we had frequently visited my uncle in the winelands, but I was not familiar with this particular farm. It turned out to be quite incredibly beautiful.

Against the backdrop of huge mountain peaks, and facing another jagged mountain in the distance, the main house stood atop a ridge, surrounded by centuries-old English oak trees and giant Chinese camphors. Decades-old vineyards blanketed the valley below, giving way to an established forest along the banks of a brook, replete with trout, and a small lake. The house – all 15 rooms of it, with its acres of garden – was flanked by old agricultural buildings, spread like a string of pearls along the ridge, nestled between gnarled oaks and ancient olive trees.

All of which is to say, I had a problem. I knew that it was *wrong* that people like me still lived in graceful Cape-Dutch manor houses on grand estates, estates that were, in effect, stolen from the indigenous inhabitants and then developed on the backs of slaves trafficked from the East.* All of this felt wrong to me not

---

* For some reason, the 17th- and 18th-century governors of the Cape Colony considered it fine to dispossess indigenous hunter-gatherers and nomadic pastoralists of their ancestral lands, annihilating their economies and cultures,

only philosophically but also in a very concrete way. As a direct result of this history, the descendants of those dispossessed local people and those dislocated slaves (the slaves who literally built my home) were *still* living on 'my' land, in relative poverty, and, not to put too fine a point on it, at my mercy. It was up to me to decide whom to employ and whom not. If I didn't hire some individual, it was unlikely that any of my neighbours would do so, since the people living on my farm were considered to be 'Solms's people'. My neighbouring landowners had their own equivalent communities living on their farms: their own people, as it were.

This does not exactly duplicate the feudal arrangements by which my German ancestors ruled their state countries, since the tenant families living on my land are nominally free citizens. Even so, the transmission across centuries of a certain way of life (especially on the old farms, where the same families have lived together for generations) can seem inevitable. Perhaps this applies not only to people like me and mine. A good case can be made that the whole of humanity is currently sleep-walking into a new form of feudalism, a 'technofeudalism', in which we all become tenants of the platforms owned by a handful of oligarchs.[11]

Freud would have had much to say about the group psychology underlying this particular manifestation of mass hypnosis, little of it comforting. On his view, hierarchy is unavoidable. He saw the 'Oedipus complex' as a kind of innate disposition to patterns of patriarchal domination. But if history keeps bending itself into the same shapes, what possible need could be served by my pious feeling that it should be otherwise? What good was my sense of wrongness? Let's be realistic here: some things never change. Why not just enjoy the beauty of the place, its generosity of scale, the gentle ambience of age? It had been this way for hundreds of years.

---

but improper to enslave them. So, they brought in slaves from outside the colony to develop the land. For the record, I am aware that it would be more correct to speak of 'enslaved people' than 'slaves', but the latter term is less cumbersome.

You only need to glance at history to know that it could have been this way forever.

More than anything else, psychoanalysis has taught me that we *resist* acknowledging pangs of conscience. We defend ourselves against them. This means that, alongside everything else that maintains the unequal structure of our societies, *feelings* have a part to play. We avoid our feelings of guilt and shame and fear of retribution by deploying *defence mechanisms*.

It was under a cloud of such feelings that, 25 years ago, after the formal ending of Apartheid and the first democratic elections, I prepared for my return to South Africa. On one of my preparatory visits, I set aside a Saturday to meet with the seven extended families who lived on the farm, allocating one hour per tenant family. My plan was to introduce myself to them and to say that, although I might look like my predecessors, I was not like them: we would from now onwards align our lives on this farm with the 'rainbow nation' values of the new South Africa. I therefore wanted to know how these families thought we could set about doing this. Unlike me, they had lived on the farm all their lives, and were therefore obviously in a better position to identify what most urgently needed to be done.

In each of those seven meetings, my introductory spiel was greeted with silence. The family members looked at each other, and at the floor, shuffling in their chairs, clearly wanting to get out of my gigantic house as quickly as possible. A little nonplussed, I introduced some reforms just as they occurred to me. I renovated their accommodation, and improved their employment contracts. In fact, I *introduced* employment contracts; previously, there had been none. Before my arrival, on rainy days when work was impossible, nobody got paid. And it rains quite a lot during Cape winters.

The workers' reaction to these innovations surprised me as much as their silence had done. People started leaving work early, especially on Fridays, and arriving late, especially on Mondays, and sometimes not arriving at all. Some came to work drunk. Things started going missing; first little things, here and there, and then more substantial items, such as a large water pump located on a riverbank, used for irrigating the vineyards. It soon occurred to me that the workers had decided I was a fool. If I didn't realize that I was in charge, they would make hay while the sun shone.

I became annoyed. Clearly, these people were taking advantage of me, taking my generosity for weakness. I considered how best to reassert my dominance. Please note the 'these people'; I was beginning to think like any other racist white South African farmer. In short, I was being put in my place. It was absurd to think that I could escape the weight of this history. The story of my farm – like that of the country as a whole – showed that we were not on the same side. Our history was one in which somebody was *always* taking advantage of somebody else. If I, fool that I was, wouldn't take advantage of the tenant workers, they would take advantage of me. For generations they'd been ruled by fear. Since they didn't need to fear me, they would do whatever they liked.

There is an old anecdote about a senior psychoanalyst who admonishes a junior candidate: 'Don't just do something, stand there.' Beware the compulsion to act. If you don't understand what's going on – especially when your lack of insight is accompanied by strong feelings – it is best to wait.

In medicine, when dealing with a condition that you don't understand, you generally begin by *taking a history*. You want to know when and how the symptoms began, under what circumstances, over what time period, and so on. The aim is to arrive at a diagnosis. Via the diagnosis, you identify the *cause* of the symptoms, and then you treat that. In psychoanalysis, the situation is no different, except that the history-taking in many respects *is* the treatment. I don't mean to imply that I was the doctor in this situation and the workers were the patient. We all needed help. Our way of relating to each other was the patient. As Samuel Shem wrote in his wonderful (1978) medical satire: when dealing with a case of cardiac arrest, the first procedure is to take your own pulse.

To help us recover the past of the farm and learn what had brought us to such a sorry pass, we hired a team of archaeologists. With the assistance of the tenant workers, they literally dug the place up. We excavated the foundations of the first buildings, trying to identify the location of the slave bell. We peeled back the stratified layers of the floor of my old wine fermentation cellar, which was built in stages between 1690 and 1831 and which housed the slaves at night. We carefully dredged a very old well, located near the cellar, searching for artefacts that might have been tossed into it. I hired a team of historians too. One of them spent months in the Cape archives, dredging up every shred of paperwork that might shed light on events that had taken place on my farm since the 1680s. Others took oral histories from the farmworkers, who remembered Apartheid all too well – and were governed by it still in their lived 'transferences'.

In a vague way, of course, I already knew the history of the Cape Colony. That is not the same as being confronted with material and documentary evidence of what happened on my own patch of land. Here, in my garden, in the mid-1700s, a slave from Bengal was burned at the stake on the mere *suspicion* of arson. Another slave – born on my farm – was going to have her children taken away and sold upcountry, due to the embarrassing fact that they were sired by the landowner's son, and he had now reached marrying age. This was in the early 1800s, after the Colony had been transferred from Dutch to British rule. The new governor had established a 'slave protectors' office'. So, the woman went there to plead her children's case. It took her two days to walk over the mountain. She provided evidence that the owner's son had promised her that their children would be free citizens.

The protector heard her out, then ruled that the boy had had no right to make such pledges. The slave was his father's property, not his; therefore the children could indeed be sold. And so they were. She probably never saw them again.

As this history emerged, piece by appalling piece, the power dynamics between the workers and me began to change. It no longer felt as if I was offering them something. It felt like I owed them something. When the research and the excavations were completed, we had been confronted with many such horrors perpetrated by my predecessors in title. We had also uncovered abundant archaeological evidence of the hunter-gatherers who lived here long before my family, up to 6,000 years ago. A Stone Age settlement had stood just 100 metres from my front door, overlapping the foundations of the first settlers' homestead. They too, like the slaves, were the ancestors of the present-day tenant workers. Holding up a beautiful microlithic stone blade from this site, the worker who discovered it remarked: 'You see, Professor: my people were here before yours.'

And there we had it. Our diagnosis. He might as well have said, 'Please explain to me again why I work for you, not the other way around? Why, exactly, is this farm yours, not ours?' The illness that beset us was a direct result of the theft of the land. This, in turn, made it clear what the treatment should be. I must return these ill-gotten gains.

At this point, the defence mechanisms kicked in. It wasn't *I* who took the land – that happened more than 300 years ago. And it wasn't taken from *these* inhabitants, of the present-day farm. And it couldn't now be divided up into 180 little parcels, one for each of us. And so on: reason after reason for maintaining the status quo. Analysis teaches you to pay attention to your true feelings, especially to the unwelcome ones, and to notice how you try to avoid them. In my case, I was employing the defence mechanism called 'rationalization': I was trying to argue my way out of what I felt to be true. Noticing this obliged me to face it. Despite my professed desire to be different from my predecessors – to do the right thing – the simple, shameful fact was that I didn't want to give the land back. I wanted to keep it, and to pass it down to my children.

At a Sunday school lesson many years ago, the teacher gave each member of the class Christmas presents: one shiny toy car or a pretty doll each, allocated as you would expect in a white South African church in the mid-1960s. She then informed the class that we should 'love thy neighbour as thyself'. Which of us would volunteer to return our presents, so that they could be given to more needy children?

I must have been about five years old, and I couldn't get my head around this crazy philosophy. Why would anyone feel the same about their neighbour as about themselves? You feel your own feelings. You couldn't feel anyone else's, so why would you prioritize theirs over yours? What mattered to you had to matter to you; what mattered to other people had to matter to those other people, surely, each one with their own concerns. And what business of mine were theirs?

For many years, well into my teens and beyond, I toyed with this sense of incoherence as if it were a riddle. If we had to be told that we *should* care about them, presumably we were free to choose not to, otherwise there would be no need to talk us into it. And if we were loving our neighbours just to get ourselves into heaven, as seemed to be the ultimate aim of our religious instruction, were we really loving our neighbours at all?

Strangely enough, in the end it was Freud who helped me out of this pit, though more by his example than his doctrines. In the material that I added to the *Revised Standard Edition*, there are many instances of Freud living by high ideals, not only as a truth-loving scientist (for which he paid dearly) but also as a social being. Consider, for example, the compassionate letter that he wrote to the mother of a gay man, quoted previously. Consider also his defence of homosexual doctors applying to train as psychoanalysts: Ernest Jones (then President of the International Psychoanalytical Association) wrote to Freud in 1921 suggesting that these applicants should be rejected as a 'general maxim', on the grounds that 'to the world it is an abhorrent crime, the committal of which by one of our members would certainly discredit us seriously'. Freud's reply was that he 'cannot agree':

That is, we cannot exclude such persons in principle, for the same reasons that we cannot condone their legal prosecution. We believe that a decision in such cases should depend on an individual examination of the other qualities of the candidate.[12]

I have already mentioned briefly Freud's defence of women's rights in the context of marriage law reform and his campaigning for the legalization of contraception in Catholic Austria. These were not popular causes, as is demonstrated by the contrast with Jones's moral cowardice. Freud's ideals are revealed also by the following letter, which he wrote spontaneously and privately to a Vienna city councillor in the winter of 1931, during widespread unemployment in the city:

> I take the liberty of proposing a procedure which could be described as *daily self-taxation of those in work*. I pledge myself, as an example, to forfeit for purposes of the 'Winter Aid' an amount of 20 Schillings from the earnings of every day [. . .] Of course, what a single citizen of no great means can achieve may be insignificant. However, if my proposal seems viable to you, please treat it as your own and recommend it to the public. Your great influence will hopefully induce many others to take up the suggestion to contribute in this manner.[13]

So much for Freud's attacking the very fabric of society. As for replacing religion with a selfish 'therapy culture' and his abhorrence of group identification, I will limit myself to one further quotation. On the occasion of the 40th anniversary of the Vienna chapter of the B'nai B'rith, a Jewish society that Freud joined in 1897 (in deeply antisemitic times), he wrote the following. He had attended fewer and fewer meetings over the years, and stopped attending completely when he fell ill with cancer. This was written in 1935:

> Since I stopped attending your meetings, the sense of belonging with you has not abated. It has kept alive the far-reaching

consensus of cultural and humanitarian ideals, as well as the (equally pleasant) affirmation of being Jewish and of Jewish origin. There is nothing more to be done for me; I am nearly twice as old as our 'Vienna [chapter]'. But with you, a Society which can always be rejuvenated once more, our community will keep faith.[14]

In case you find Freud's position confusing, he drew a sharp distinction between Jewish identity and Jewish religion: 'Although a good Jew who has never repudiated Judaism, I cannot overlook the fact that my absolutely negative attitude to all religion, including the Jewish one, separates me from most of our kin.'[15]

I don't recall whether I returned my toy car or not that Christmas. If I did, I suspect I wasn't happy about it. Only much later did I grasp what I now take to be the meaning of this Sunday School injunction, to love your neighbour as you love yourself. Each of us is the centre of our own universe. Yet we can't live as solipsists, each of us in glorious isolation, the only light in the universe. To a surprising degree, almost all of our emotional drives seem aimed at influencing the feelings of others. Lust wishes to stimulate lust: we desire to be desired. Likewise, attachment seeks to foster attachment, and play playfulness. Rage strives to strike fear. Even fear shrinks us to elicit mercy, a gateway drug to care. All of these feelings seem to require the feelings of others for their satisfaction. Who among us doesn't want our neighbour to love us – to care about and appreciate and *know* us for who we actually are? Perhaps this seems trivial and obvious, but it goes deep. Without any feeling for the feelings of others – without *empathy* – we can never get what we really want.

This has many implications. For example, rather than condemn violence as a negative tendency that must be wiped off the face of society, perhaps it should be understood as the expression of an innate human need: the need to get rid of frustrating obstacles and impediments; that is, to deal aggressively with things that deny the satisfaction of one's needs. Where would we be, biologically speaking, if we didn't have a drive to stake our claims upon the available resources and then to defend those claims against others? Where we see anger, we could try to recognize what it *means*. This is easier said than done, but it becomes very important in unequal societies such as South Africa. Here, as with the other drives, we cannot (and shouldn't try to) get rid of the need itself; all we can do is to learn how best to satisfy it. The innate instinctual behaviour called 'affective attack' is not always the best way to remove frustrating obstacles and impediments in life. But we need to recognize the meaning – and the value – of the feeling of anger itself.

And not only anger; all feelings. This brings me back to my uncomfortable realization that, in truth, I didn't want to give my farm back. There is nothing wrong with self-interest, I now thought to myself, so long as you take account of the fact that *everybody else has self-interest too*. Self-interest needn't imply selfish interest. So, the problem became: how can I play fairly? How can I preserve my own interest while simultaneously taking account of the equivalent self-interest of the tenant workers? How can I love my neighbour as myself, without loving them more than myself?

Once you face the avoided facts, you get your problem-solving mind back. The solution that presented itself was this. Together with a like-minded friend and neighbour, with whom I had deep discussions about these things while my farm was being excavated, we mortgaged our two properties in order to secure a large bank loan. This loan we used to purchase the farm adjacent to ours for the workers and their families. They became the beneficiaries of a trust, set up to take ownership of the third farm, which was just as large and every bit as beautiful as our two farms were. That way, my friend and I got to keep our historic farms, while we simultaneously enabled the resident workers to become landowners, too. Of course, we had to ensure that the workers' farm was economically sustainable, because we were on the line for it. So, we formed a partnership: each of us – the neighbour, the trust and I – took an equal share in a company that farmed the three properties, which were leased to the company. Now we all had a stake in the success of each other's farms.

We also set up a museum: a site of conscience, in which the true story of what happened on this land was told. Among other things, every slave who gave their life to its development is memorialized by name on granite plaques which cover one of the walls of the museum.*

Our partnership wasn't the end of the workers' troubles or my own, by any means. In the years that followed, we faced many challenges, including some very serious ones, and we still do. Not least among these has been an ongoing 'return of the repressed': our mistrust of each other, and the attendant automatized tendency to take advantage of each other. We have been forced to confront many defences that we have erected along the way. In my case, they included the manic belief that Nelson Mandela died for our sins, meaning that we were all forgiven, coupled with something of a white-messiah complex, by which means I sought to exempt myself from the guilt that all beneficiaries of colonialism and slavery and Apartheid must bear.

The truth is that my quality of life and that of my children still is much better than that of the tenant workers and their families. Therefore, they still have reason to be angry. So, there is work yet to be done.

'It is impossible', Freud wrote in 1930, 'to overlook the extent to which civilization is built up upon a renunciation of drive'.[16] This view follows naturally from his conception of drive:† not only

---

* Where a name could be discovered. If it couldn't, they were memorialized by a plaque dedicated to an 'unknown female slave', as the case may be, together with whatever other demographic information we could find.

† To be clear, my own conception is slightly different from Freud's: we cannot renounce our drives, we can only renounce our instinctual responses to them. The great task of mental life (and of civilization) is the development of better predictions as to how to satisfy our drives, and to reconcile them with each other, and with the drives of others.

from the compulsive and relentless pleasure-seeking of the libido, but likewise from the blind destructiveness of rage. Since there seems no real alternative to living in civilization, it follows that all we can hope to achieve with psychoanalysis is to 'replace neurotic misery with common unhappiness'.[17] There is no such thing as a conflict-free existence.

Is this really the best we can hope for? The development of neuroscience over the past half century gives us one great advantage over Freud. We now understand, in a way that he could not, that we are animated by multiple emotional values, and one of these is very strikingly not like the others.

Let me explain. For all that they are usually *directed* at others, fear, attachment, play and so on all register to a greater or lesser extent as our own impulses, serving our own biological needs. Even lust tends to be experienced as a somewhat selfish drive for pleasure, though it is generally mediated by pragmatism, if not any deeper concern with the welfare of others.* Yet one of our emotional drives seems as close to pure altruism as anything in biology. This is the drive to nurture, to *care* for our offspring.

The prototype of care is raising a child: a complex task that clearly requires an astoundingly open-ended and flexible range of behaviours. Once triggered, the caring instinct can be engaged for years on end, if not for the rest of your life. It involves doing much or all of what one would do to sustain oneself, on behalf of another, for as long as it takes. Think of the life-support system for a body in coma. Think of the nurses on my ward.

---

* Indeed, the idea that someone might have sex for reasons other than their own sensual desire tends to strike us as a bad thing: the weight of popular opinion on sex work, for example, seems to be distributed along a continuum from 'terrible injustice' to 'somewhat regrettable fact of life', with takers for 'it's good, actually' remaining rare. We seem to find the idea of anyone having sex for reasons other than pleasure (or biological reproduction) vaguely immoral. Even sex for purely altruistic reasons may strike us as somehow a betrayal of the true purpose of it. I need hardly add that nonconsensual sex *is* immoral.

Care also drives the human version of nesting: an impulse to secure the environment of the object of nurture, both from physical threats and from unsettling social and emotional forces. It is to this end that we must procure financial and other resources. To a great extent, it is care that makes us go to work.

As an instinct, it is surprisingly promiscuous. It invests us not only in the fate of our own young, but also that of other people and other species, and even inanimate objects that evoke an impression of sentient vulnerability. (It doesn't take much to evoke such impressions; a rich seam in psychology research involves videos of small oval objects that we reliably interpret, with concern, as being 'under attack' from large triangular ones.) It is via care, too, that questions of altruism and legacy meet, since the world that we leave behind is the one in which our descendants must live.

In my clinical work I have seen how parents respond when their children become ill or disabled. There is almost nothing they will not sacrifice for them – not infrequently, in the case of disability, for an entire lifetime. As for how parents respond to the death of a child, I would prefer not to think about that. I have witnessed it many times.

This is what Freud wrote to his bereaved son-in-law when his 27-year-old daughter Sophie died suddenly on January 25, 1920:

> You know how great our sorrow is; we know what grief you must be suffering; I make no attempt to console you, and you can do nothing for us [. . .] We can only bow our heads under the blow like the poor helpless creatures we are, mere playthings for the higher powers.[18]

It was in the wake of this loss that Freud developed his view that 'the aim of all life is death'. The timing seems significant.

Yet, even in the case of our own children, where the drive to nurture reaches its biological zenith, we do not *only* care for them and care for them *only*. There are times, often when our children are most demanding, that we find ourselves thinking: 'what about *my* needs?' This thought doesn't necessarily result in us prioritizing ourselves, but sometimes it does. Sometimes it results in less than good-enough parenting. Sometimes it results in abuse.

Inadequate parental support is not, by any means, always a moral fault on the part of parents. They too were children once, and they too may not have been adequately cared for. Social and economic factors can play a fundamental role. It is obviously very much more difficult to care adequately for your children if you don't have the practical resources and support to do so. It is therefore no accident that certain mental illnesses (and almost all the major ones) are more prevalent among those who were raised in relative poverty.

There is also the tendency for relational patterns and inadequacies to repeat themselves down the generations: a large subject that we can't go into properly here. Let me just observe that, while the drive to care is innate, how we actually go about it is something we have to learn. Generally speaking, we are no better than our teachers.

For much of his life, Freud would wake up at 7 a.m., take a quick breakfast, and then conduct clinical consultations from 8 a.m. until noon. After lunch with his family, and a few errands, he would return to his practice in the mid-afternoon, continuing consultations until dinner at 9 p.m. For the remainder of the evening, he would work, mainly writing up clinical observations and maintaining his voluminous correspondence, often staying up until 1 a.m. He maintained this exhausting schedule for decades. He once said that psychoanalysis is 'a cure by love'.[19] If you've ever been a therapist, looking down a full day's slate of appointments, you will appreciate just how much *energy* all this curing by love must have cost him. How strange that he has been painted as a barbarian at the gate.

Whatever the reasons for mental troubles in any individual case, I have been arguing in this book that the only way to treat their *causes* is to help each patient find better ways of meeting their emotional needs. This requires psychotherapy. Psychotherapy could be described as a 're-parenting' process. It takes time and effort. That is, it requires care.

Our duty of care to psychiatric patients requires us to do more than give them pills. As the evidence abundantly shows, psychopharmacological and other physical treatments merely suppress psychiatric symptoms, incompletely and with side effects. Those treatments do not and cannot cure mental illness. For a cure to be achieved, in all but the simplest of acute cases, the patient must go through the arduous process of re-learning how to meet their emotional needs. There is no other way. To claim otherwise is, I believe, to mislead our patients.

This is not to imply that most psychiatrists are liars when they prescribe medication. Most of them no doubt sincerely think they are treating disorders that are caused by 'chemical imbalances'. Still, the evidence is very clear. If they think they are prescribing a cure, they are fooling themselves as much as their patients.

Where could such self-deception come from? I have tried to show that it stems from the illusion that we can or should have a physiological psychiatry; that there need not be any real distinction between psychiatry and neurology. Meynert was under the spell of this illusion when he claimed that 'treatment of the soul' implies 'more than we can accomplish'.

But his claim can be interpreted in another way. It could be read as saying that it is *too difficult* to treat the soul, that it requires more care than we are willing to invest. I don't think this is what Meynert meant, but I do believe it is the other main source of our self-deception. Here I mean our self-deception as a society. If psychotherapy is akin to re-parenting, then it seems that we as a society are not willing to put the necessary time and effort and money into *the children of other people*. We are unwilling to love our neighbours as ourselves. So we deceive ourselves – and allow governments and big pharmaceutical companies and health insurance schemes to deceive us – into believing that you can mend the course of entire human lives through the simple administration of pills. We buy into an anti-psychoanalytical culture that claims that one can fix a life quickly and easily and cheaply.

I am not blameless in this. I recognize just how hard it is, not only from my own case, but also from my decades of working as a psychoanalyst, trying to change the lives of others, one life at a time. Nowadays I find myself increasingly reluctant when taking on new patients. I don't turn them away, but I am more aware of the struggles that lie ahead of me. As I get to know each patient, and forge an alliance with the part of them that is willing to face the difficult facts about themselves, my reluctance gives way to renewed determination: to help them stay the course when the going gets tough. In the end, the rewards are considerable. To witness, in case after case, how the pattern of a whole life *can* be changed, and to know that I have helped, is deeply satisfying. But it would be pointless to pretend that it's easy.

Psychoanalysis is a cure wrought by loving your neighbour as yourself. You need only recognize that your patient is suffering just as you have suffered, or might have suffered, had things gone wrong for you in the way that they did for this person. There is an infinite number of things that can go wrong in a life. Sometimes they go very badly wrong. Helping patients to find their way back to viable trajectories requires not only a lot of work but also an ongoing willingness to remain in contact with your own bloodier places.

None of us is exempt from the task of learning to meet our basic needs, and to reconcile them with each other, and with the needs of the other selves that share our milieu: first in the family, then on the playground, and then in the wider world. You must find other selves to love and to love you, both affectionately and sexually; you must make friends and achieve status in groups that you can call your own; you must fend off rivals and fight the baddies (for there always are baddies); and you must stay safe while doing so. In addition, you must engage with and explore the endless unknowns; until, at last, you begin to understand, and, with luck, acquire a modicum of wisdom.

Looking back over my decades of involvement with psychoanalysis, I believe I can honestly recommend it as a way of thinking and working and being. There's something very powerful about the notion that, simply by attending closely to the feelings and memories of another person – the seemingly inconsequential details of a life – we can gain insights not only into their inner worlds, but into the deep structure of *all* souls. Each of us contains the secret truth of all of us. And as I have found in my lifetime working in Freud's long shadow, there is always more to discover.

So let me urge the scientists and practitioners and caring souls of the future: take up the struggle for what we might call a psychoanalytic culture, not only in science and psychiatry but also in our societies. As Freud once wrote to Einstein, reflecting toward the end of his life upon the uncertain standing of the discipline he had created:

> Admittedly, it is not altogether a matter of regret that one has opted for psychology. There is no greater, richer, more mysterious subject, worthy of every effort of the human intellect, than the life of the mind.[20]

EPILOGUE
The Cause

It seemed significant that Teddy P's mental collapse occurred after a separation and a bereavement. From my experience of working with depression, I'd expected him to relate a history of dreadful childhood separations and losses, as is common in children who later become depressed. Yet, to my slight surprise, nothing very dramatic seemed to have happened in his early years.

His parents were unhappily married. His father, a bookkeeper, played rather a small role in this story. At weekends, and in the evenings after work, he forfeited the company of his wife and children in favour of the pub. Teddy remembered him with indifference as an absent figure, but not especially negative in any sense.

Teddy's mother stayed at home and spent her time chain-smoking in the kitchen. She took him and his older brother with her when she went to the shops or visited her friends, but he felt very acutely that she never engaged with her children in an emotional way. She somehow seemed uninterested in them as psychological beings. Teddy remembered her always watching television or listening to the radio. In his descriptions, there was also a note of revulsion: he called her obese, and reported disgusting odours and sounds emanating from the lavatory when she was in there. (I wondered why he was waiting at the door.)

Despite his wish to be more engaged with her, or more likely because this wish was thwarted, Teddy's revulsion suggested hostility as well as longing. More than a century ago, Freud drew our attention to this *ambivalence* towards a longed-for person, which is so common in depression. Freud supposed that the hostility gets deflected inwards – *I* am bad – resulting in the self-loathing that is so typical of depressed patients.

He would have found much to note in Teddy's experience of toilet training. As a young boy, Teddy suffered more than usually from incontinence. It was obvious to him, as a toddler, that his mother got annoyed whenever he needed help to go to the bathroom. He therefore held on for as long as he could, leading to accidents, which of course irritated her even more. He remembered feeling constantly ashamed: not only unloved but unlovable.

There is a cliché about analysis that it entails little more than moaning about the time that you didn't get the pony you wanted. Well, sometimes the way a patient fixates upon not getting a pony points to something more profound.

Research shows that early bereavement is less associated with depression than is the tantalizing presence of an emotionally unavailable parent.[1] Impoverished communities, similarly, are more distressed by their circumstances when they live in close proximity to advantaged ones, as frequently happens in South Africa.

Despite the unspectacular nature of the facts I have described so far, it's interesting that both Teddy P and his brother developed significant psychiatric problems. This suggests to me that something systematic was at work in the emotional climate of their childhood.

At the age of 15, Teddy's brother made a serious suicide attempt and was hospitalized. Teddy remembered visiting him at a residential psychiatric ward once a week with their parents. He was impressed by the atmosphere of attentive concern that surrounded his brother, speculating to me that this could have been what first gave him the idea of studying medicine. He was nine.

Understandably worried, Teddy's parents took their sons to a string of guidance clinics and psychiatrists over the next few years, but, though they followed the advice they were given, nothing seemed to change. Eventually, when Teddy reached 14, his parents split up. He suffered his first depressive collapse two years later, ending up, like his brother, in hospital. There he received medication and a brief course of therapy, before returning to school with a new outlook, obtaining excellent grades. True to his childhood inspiration, he went off to study medicine.

It was shortly after qualifying as a doctor that he got involved with the girlfriend with whom he experienced the sexual problems described at the start of this book. Combined with the death of his mother, her rejection of Teddy dented his self-esteem and eventually affected his working life dramatically. We know the rest: depression and panic attacks, nonepileptic seizures, multiple drug prescriptions, and complications resulting from their many side effects and interactions.

With the support of the referring neurologist, I recommended three sessions a week of psychotherapy. Teddy was still unemployed when we started his treatment, but most of his medications were being withdrawn and he was more lucid than before. On the downside, he was also increasingly anxious and depressed, and very unsure that quitting his drugs was a good idea. As if to prove it, he produced three more seizures in the first two months of our therapy, followed by visits to the casualty department of my hospital. My fear that I had missed something was allayed by a chat with Teddy's neurologist. She thought that, while it was possible that these seizures were withdrawal symptoms, they were much more likely to be 'functional', like the earlier ones. Either way, they certainly weren't epilepsy. Adult-onset seizures, she reminded me, are always symptomatic of something else.

For the most part Teddy's depression presented in standard ways: chronic low mood, dark thoughts, hopelessness, lack of energy, self-criticism. He slept through most of his days and withdrew almost entirely from company, apart from occasional visits from an aunt. One unusual aspect of his presentation, however, was indecisiveness. Actually, that's not quite the right word: he had enormous difficulty formulating and expressing *opinions* about anything to anyone. He just agreed with whatever the person he was talking to said, to the point that he found himself agreeing with starkly opposing viewpoints from one interaction to the next, on the political events of the day and the controversies that rumbled within his remaining family alike. They were all the same to him.

My clinical formulation was equally standard: as a child, Teddy had felt rage towards his frustratingly indifferent and emotionally unavailable mother, but still he longed desperately for her love. He resolved this conflict by shutting down his aggression and assertiveness toward her, to the point of relinquishing all agency. This childish solution to his emotional problems, which left him feeling terribly bad about himself, had the dubious benefit that his extended family was now being *forced* to care for him, much as his parents had been forced to attend to his incontinence. (Freud called this 'gain from illness'.)

I put the suggestion to Teddy, and he agreed that it made sense. I tried not to put too much weight on that, though. He would agree with anything.

As the treatment progressed, more memories returned, often in a distinctive way. Teddy would allude to something as if we had discussed it in an earlier session. I would indicate that this was new information, and he would blink, puzzled for a moment, before backing down and saying he was sure I was right. This naturally made me much less certain of my own memory. After the session I would check over my notes, and every time, it was indeed new information to me.

I wondered whether Teddy was conflating this course of therapy with his earlier one. His mind was, after all, still quite hazy. Then again, blurring past and present is exactly what 'transference' is all about. Perhaps he thought I couldn't be angry with him for something if I thought I was already meant to know it – an understandable stratagem among children of distracted caregivers. Or perhaps he imagined that I, the figure of authority and care in this situation, should know by intuition what was clogging up his insides and causing him such discomfort. It was as if these scraps of his history spontaneously leaked out, and it was my fault for not catching them earlier; as if I should have known that he needed the bathroom.

Here was one such revelation. Teddy mentioned in passing, as if it was common knowledge between us, that the woman he started dating after medical school had been a fellow patient in the psychiatric clinic where he was admitted as a teenager. She had remained in contact with him ever since. When I said that he hadn't mentioned this before, he was surprised.

The more I learnt about this girlfriend, the clearer it became that she was a very unsuitable choice. She was being treated for a severe personality disorder when they met. Before she dumped him, she emptied his bank account. He didn't report the crime to anyone.

Here is a second revelation that Teddy made as if we had already been discussing it, though it was new to me. His teenage hospitalization followed an incident at a sleepover in which he fondled the penis of a sleeping friend. He was very ashamed of this. When I suggested that it might have been somewhat consensual, since it was unlikely that his friend would have stayed asleep through it, Teddy became reluctant. He seemed to want to contradict me, but of course he found that difficult. At length he explained that the psychotherapist at the clinic where he received in-patient treatment had helped him precisely by getting him to accept that he was a paedophile.

This seemed strange. How can a teenager fondling another teenager be described as a paedophile? When I questioned it, Teddy insisted that it made sense to him. In fact, it was precisely by facing this ugly truth about himself, and sticking to a list of strict prohibitions that his therapist had given him (no television or internet in the evenings; only dinner, study and sleep) that he managed to pull himself together, turn his grades around and become the doctor I saw before me.

I was at a loss. Clearly Teddy had found something useful in this diagnosis. Still, I didn't understand it. Perhaps the therapist had said 'homosexual' rather than 'paedophile' – but that didn't make sense either, since Teddy seemed pretty thoroughly straight.

The only sense I could make of it was that it gave him another opportunity to dislike himself: *I am bad*.

It was around this point that he first mentioned, again in the guise of recapping old information, an unrequited crush on a girl at school. She shared his science classes (this was before the incident at the sleepover). Teddy couldn't stop thinking about her. He stalked her on social media and sent her increasingly desperate messages, none of which received a response. Teddy became more insistent, bombarding her into the night with pleas and demands, until she blocked him. At this point he began following her home in the evenings, stalking her physically. This, I thought, was clear evidence of his aggression towards unavailable love objects.

The girl's parents told Teddy's mother that if she didn't remove him from the school, they would seek a restraining order. Humiliated and terrified, Teddy stopped going to classes, but still spent his nights trawling social media looking for images of this girl, to which he would masturbate compulsively. The self-loathing he developed over this time was so intense that he contemplated suicide.

A short while later, following the incident at the sleepover (another boundary violation), he experienced the crisis that landed him in hospital.

It seemed fairly obvious to me that the friend somehow stood in for the girl. When I put this to Teddy, he agreed. Of course he did.

Fortunately, there were other signs that we were on the right track. With his aggression coming gradually into the open, he suffered no further seizures. His depression started to lift. He was allowed to drive again. He started to venture out of his apartment, spending several hours each day in a nearby library. He became friendly with one of the librarians.

I should point out that everything in Teddy's story so far is compatible with the classical Freudian conception of depression: namely, that it arises through the deflection inward of aggressive impulses felt originally toward a lost love object. Freud took such love for a maternal object to be literally a form of sexual desire ('oral libido'). But despite this support from classical theory, and the apparently good results achieved by my predecessor's diagnosis of early-onset paedophilia, I still wasn't convinced that Teddy's problem was sexual at root. There was too much that didn't make sense. We needed a smoking gun.

On this note, the relationship with the librarian became a significant area of concern. Teddy said he was becoming attracted to her. He courted her with free medical advice, and then free medications, including large quantities of opiates. I thought she was taking advantage of him, just as his previous girlfriend had done, but I also worried about the ethics of his own behaviour. The themes of unsuitable choices and boundary violations struck me again, just as they did in his stories about the sleeping friend and the girl he followed home from school.

Teddy seemed not to have the emotional equipment to hold anything back. It was as if, once a channel of intimacy had opened up, he compulsively voided himself into it. Images of jellyfish and flatworms entered my mind, boneless creatures that transact all their vital business through a single aperture. Freud, of course, thought that the growing embryo retraces its own evolutionary history. That turned out to be false, yet it's true that we all start life as organisms with a single opening. It's called the blastopore, the first gateway between the inner and outer worlds. Couldn't Teddy's one channel be a starting point, too, for an emotional constitution more suited to its purpose?

About eight months into the therapy, he had almost no money left. His relatives were losing patience. He started talking about applying for jobs, but never seemed to get around to it. I interpreted this as a defence, noting that it allowed him to remain dependent, which is what he fundamentally wanted – his family standing in for his mother. It might be argued that sponging off relatives is simply a form of laziness, not requiring any further explanation, but I suggest that this overlooks both his willingness to do hard work and the self-defeating quality of Teddy's behaviour. It should be clear by now that he craved love intensely, and could become frankly relentless when it was withheld from him, always ending in self-loathing. Yet here he was again, pushing his last allies to breaking point.

Around this time, Teddy retrieved a very early memory. This one wasn't a fact that he said he had already mentioned. It was something emotionally charged and upsetting, something he seemed surprised to find welling up within himself.

When he was small, his bedroom had been adjacent to his parents' bedroom, and he was painfully aware of the fact that his mother was just a few feet away. Only the wall separated them. His desire to be with her was so frenzied that he lay in bed wanting to scratch through the wall with his nails.

I made a link between this urge and his uninvited touching of the sleeping friend's penis, and before that, his stalking of the girl at school. Teddy's eyes shone. Yes, they were all the same, touched by the same desperation and shame. He could see it. Rage, too, I suggested. The thought made him uncomfortable, but he didn't disagree.

His forgetfulness and vagueness seemed to be lifting in chronological order, backward through the mists: from the uninvited touching to the stalking to the burrowing through walls. Though not by any means a rule, this pattern is common, and produces a satisfying sense of *getting closer*. Shortly, we shall hear of another striking case of Teddy's boundary violations, dating to his sixth year. Before that, however, I must report some troubling examples of the same thing from his adult life.

A few weeks after that session, Teddy was offered a job. The prospect of working again seemed to energize him, until his professional indemnity providers informed him that he would be on his own if he started lining up customers for cheap overseas cosmetic surgery, payment on commission. That wasn't a risk they were willing to insure.

To my surprise, he argued his obviously futile case quite vigorously. For better or worse, the very passive version of Teddy I first met was disappearing. A different set of problems were coming into view. Behind the Teddy who couldn't see any options was a Teddy who couldn't take no for an answer.

He and the librarian began dating. It became apparent that he had made another unfortunate choice. For reasons we can only guess at, this woman couldn't bear to be touched. Teddy was once again left with the same desperation he had felt in relation to his mother. The impasse dragged on for months, until the librarian finally left him, no longer willing to tolerate his pleas for affection in exchange for prescription painkillers. (She made a clean breast of it, too; I imagine she found a less complicated supplier, sources of opioids being easier to substitute than sources of love.)

At this point, my patient seemed in real danger of relapsing. The relationship on which he had been relying for so many of his emotional needs had stopped dead. Panic and grief – that is, depression – was already his habitual mode, and now it seemed a natural reaction as well. I had a feeling that something terrible was about to happen. The fact that it didn't is no particular credit to me, and perhaps not to therapy either, but it is instructive.

We need to leave Teddy alone for a moment.

Following the teenage suicide attempt and brief hospitalization, Teddy's older brother didn't manage to rally into anything like Teddy's academic success. Instead, he dropped out of school before his A-Levels, drifted through many unskilled and temporary jobs, and got involved in petty crime. After a few years of that, his girlfriend became pregnant. To everyone's surprise, he decided to stay with her: to rise to the occasion.

Very late, the pregnancy failed. Teddy wasn't in touch with his brother at the time but he remembered it as a terrible blow, resounding through their family.

Perhaps surprisingly, the couple stayed together, riding out the shock of grief. They tried again, and kept trying. It took years, but it happened for them, a miracle: a daughter. Teddy's brother was working hard to make them a home, to give his little family some stability. He trained as a locksmith and then as an electrician, soon making good money. And he had recently expressed an interest in spending time with his younger sibling. For whatever reason, he wanted to put their family back together.

Teddy was wary. His brother would want to talk about childhood memories, he said. I supposed he must be thinking of something in particular, but when I pressed him he said he didn't know what he had meant. In any case, when they did meet up at last, he found to his surprise that he enjoyed his brother's company very much. He especially liked the two-year-old daughter, his niece. He hadn't realized, he said, how much he had been missing the comforts of family and domesticity. (Comforts that he had arguably never known.) The only problem, Teddy confessed after much hesitation, was when his niece held his hand, or cuddled him, or climbed into his lap. At these moments, he was filled with a terrible fear that he would get an erection. He didn't, he hastened to add; he just couldn't shake the idea that he might. Good grief, I thought, maybe he really *is* a paedophile. I was struck by a feeling that, for all his apparent passivity, he was capable of terrible harm.

In a short time, however, it became clear that all Teddy wanted was for somebody to want him, to want to spend time with him, to answer his desperate need to be loved. He became touchingly interested in his niece's development, the vivid sense that she was already a complete little personality. I braced for any hint that he was taking advantage of her, abusing her in some way, but in his stumbling, hesitant, very uncle-like fashion, he seemed to dote on her. It was clear (clear as it ever can be) that he simply loved her.

Teddy started to chafe at the paedophile diagnosis. Without prompting, he began to theorize that his fear about inappropriate sexual associations grew out of an overflowing craving for human contact. He wanted sex, of course, but his longing for affection had become confused in his mind with sexual feelings, which were, after all, easier to name, and in certain, masculine ways more legitimate to act on.

He didn't yet seem angry about how he had been led to think of himself. I wondered if he would.

One day, he was offered a job as a proper doctor: an emergency physician.

In the days before he started, he would wake in the middle of the night, convinced that he no longer knew how to practise medicine. It was only a matter of time before his employers realized how incompetent he was, that he was a fraud – or he killed someone.

As it happened, he managed the job perfectly well – at an instrumental level at least, as his mother had done with her children. His anxiety abated. Or rather, it transferred to me. Almost immediately, he fell head over heels in love with a fellow doctor, who was both married and clearly uninterested in him. (Unsuitable choice.) He began to have violently sexual dreams about her. He followed her on social media and masturbated compulsively to pictures of her. (Boundary violation.)

To make matters worse, it emerged that he was taking all sorts of risks with his patients. He cut corners in alarming ways, and showed a striking disregard for their actual welfare. Also, he frequently spoke about them in disparaging terms. It was as if, on some level, he didn't really care what happened to any of them, that none of it was quite real to him.

When I drew Teddy's attention to this, I suggested that perhaps he had been anxious about taking the job not only because he was worried about his ability as a doctor, but also because he was aware of his habit of trying to cheat a system that was fundamentally about helping people. It didn't matter how good his knowledge was. He couldn't care for his patients unless – I could hear that I was growing hectoring and tried to ease off – he actually *cared* about them. He agreed: yes, that made sense.

So began the most moving passage of our work. It became possible to link this tendency with his other boundary violations, starting with his stalking, and continuing through the various iterations up to his current workplace infatuation. Teddy came to the view that, since he had never received proper love, from anyone really, least of all from his mother, he didn't know how to give it, not even to his patients. This insight stood in sharp contrast to what he observed, so unexpectedly, in his brother. His brother's nurturing love for his daughter was palpable, as was his affection for his younger brother, his genuine wish to have Teddy around, and likewise – most surprising of all to Teddy – the unconditional love that his niece showed him, and evoked from him. Through what amounted to an accidental baby observation, like the ones undertaken by trainee psychoanalysts, he seemed to be discovering his own caring self.

As we worked through these thoughts and feelings in our sessions, Teddy revealed more and more empathic concern for his patients. I glimpsed this when he told me about them as people (never revealing their names, of course), and expressed an ongoing concern with their lives after he had managed the initial emergency. This led me to see what I hadn't noticed before: he really was a good diagnostician, a very talented doctor.

It was during this transformative phase in the treatment that Teddy confessed the other boundary violation I mentioned previously. It happened when he was approximately five years old – since he was sure it happened before he started 'big school' at six. Again, he was under the impression that he had divulged this story to me long ago. He hadn't.

During one of those dreary childhood visits to his mother's relatives, while his brother was in the garden, Teddy had played 'doctor-doctor' with a girl cousin in her bedroom. The game culminated in him poking a finger into the little girl's vagina, which made her cry. He apologized, and begged her not to tell the adults. Apparently she didn't, but still he worried that she might have told his brother. This, perhaps, is why Teddy was reluctant to meet up with him all those years later.

How extraordinary, I thought: Teddy's very first action as a 'doctor' was the violation of a 'patient'. Perhaps this was why he had been ready to accept the label of paedophile. For a boy who sexually molests another child of the same age, it still didn't make sense as a *diagnosis*; it didn't imply a lifelong sexual fixation on minors. Teddy's behaviour could have suggested emotional problems, along the lines of his urgent wish to burrow through the wall into his mother's bedroom, but the truth is that children fairly routinely do such things with each other. Still, I could see how a judgement on such behaviour might have struck at his roots: so desperate for intimacy that he was willing to test the nascent rules; and later, so certain of his own badness that only a label associated with the utmost depravity would do to explain his shameful actions.

By now, nearly two years into the treatment, the whole transference had become clear. The reason Teddy kept falling for unavailable and unsuitable people was surely because they stood in for his mother. Their failure to reciprocate his feelings frustrated him to the point of rage, but he couldn't express that. All he knew how to do was to hound and pester, scratching at the wall to get closer. When that failed, he allowed himself to get into trouble, rather as he had used incontinence as a last resort to summon care: a dirty protest, an aggressive relinquishing of self-control that left him hating himself instead of (or at least as much as) his love object. His assumed unlovability became a self-fulfilling prophecy.

Teddy fully agreed with this understanding of why his life had fallen apart. For my part, I felt that we had established a reasonably accurate reconstruction of his development. It was neat, but not too neat. It fitted all the facts – both from his history and the new data he was generating, since of course these patterns kept repeating. That was to be expected. The difference was, now he caught himself in the act each time he felt inclined to do it again, and then changed tack. In the end, only consciousness can free us from the hold of unconscious compulsions. It takes time and patience.

Alongside this 'working through', Teddy gradually developed more satisfying ways of gaining *and giving* love. By the time that we ended his treatment, which lasted just over four years, he was engaged to a woman he had met during the inflection point of the therapy. She certainly broke the mould; a health visitor introduced to him by his brother's wife, it would be difficult to imagine a more caring person.

Teddy's depression remitted completely. From what I gather several years later, he has continued to do well. I occasionally hear reports from medical colleagues struck by what a devoted clinician he turned out to be. As far as I am aware, none of them know that I treated him.

The health service can be a judgemental world. It's not easy to return to the fray, especially after a murky period of absence that is rumoured to conceal a mental breakdown. That takes a strong person. But Teddy is one, actually. People tell me he is an outstanding doctor. Having got to know him quite well, I believe it.

Notes

INTRODUCTION: The Symptom

1. Shorter (1997).
2. See for example Joseph Bernstein's recent article in the *New York Times* (March 22, 2023) titled 'Not Your Daddy's Freud', which opens with the sentence: 'A new generation of analysts and patients is embracing the father of psychoanalysis – in magazines and memes and many hours on the couch.' See also Rachel Connolly's article in the *Financial Times* (May 12, 2023): 'I'd Never Stuck with Therapy, Then I Tried Psychoanalysis.' In an article for *Religion News* (October 5, 2023) titled 'Is it Time for Conservative Christians to Give Freud Another Look?', Jacob Lupfer writes: 'Freud's insights about parental influences and the unconscious mind may lead to deeper commitments among people who love God as father and church as mother.' See also Andrew Hartz's article in *Quillette* (September 9, 2024): 'Freud's Best Theory'; Merve Emre's reviews in *The New Yorker* (June 3 & 10, 2024): 'What Does Freud Still Have to Teach Us?: Come for the Oedipus Complex; Stay for the Later Troubled Musings on the Fate of Humanity' and 'Subconsciously Yours: Does Every Generation Get the Freud They Deserve?'; Jacqueline Rose's article in *The Guardian* (October 10, 2024): 'What Sigmund Freud can Teach us about the Middle East and #MeToo'; David Stromberg's article in *The Hedgehog Review* (November 13, 2024): 'War, Death, and Intellectualism: Freud and the Limits of Analysis'; and there are many more.
3. Auden, W. H. (1940), 'In Memory of Sigmund Freud'.
4. Nagel (1974).
5. Freud (1927), p. 52.

CHAPTER ONE: Censors

1. Broca (1861).
2. Kleist (1934).
3. Luria & Majovski (1977), p. 963.
4. Luria was born on July 16, 1902. Freud's first letter to him was dated July 3, 1922.

5   Luria (1979) tells us that he filled notebooks with her free associations, but there is no evidence that he wrote a report of the case.
6   Luria (1940), p. 510.
7   Luria (1979), pp. 23–4.
8   Luria (1973), pp. 341–2.
9   E.g., Lobner & Levitan (1978), Kozulin (1984), Miller (1998).
10 Van der Veer & Valsiner (1991), p. 78.
11 Ibid, p. 22.
12 Kozulin (1984), p. 20.
13 Pappenheim (1990), p. 5.
14 Valkanova (2016), p. 14.
15 Kozulin (1984), p. 1.
16 Ibid., p. 89.
17 Joravsky (1974), p. 24.
18 Cole (1979), p. 198. Cole made similar remarks to me personally, in a letter dated April 1, 1989.
19 Letter dated March 17, 1987.
20 Mecacci (1988), pp. 268–9. Mecacci made similar remarks to me personally, in a letter dated March 24, 1992.
21 Freud (1895), p. 143.
22 Popper (1934), p. 86.
23 Pauli seems to have first uttered these words in the late 1940s. See https://www.math.columbia.edu/~woit/wordpress/?p=13455
24 Frankfurt (2005), p. 33.
25 Popper (1963), p. 35.
26 Letter dated February 8, 1934.
27 Skinner (1953), p. 160.

CHAPTER TWO: The Interpretation of Dreams

1   Feinstein et al. (2011).
2   Ibid.
3   Dement & Kleitman (1957).
4   Jouvet (1965).
5   McCarley & Hobson (1977), p. 1219.
6   Hobson & McCarley (1977), pp. 1346, 1338.
7   Ibid., p. 1338.
8   Solms (1997, 2000).
9   Olds & Milner (1954).
10 Sulloway (1979).
11 Freud (1882), p. 39.

NOTES 279

12 Freud (2012 [1885–7]), pp. 78–89.
13 Freud (1888), p. 690.
14 Freud (1891), p. 54; emphasis added.
15 Ibid., p. 55.
16 Freud (1893), pp. 195–6.
17 Freud (1912), p. 259.
18 Popper (1974), p. 985.
19 Kant (1784).

CHAPTER THREE: The Mental Apparatus

1 See Freud (1882). Freud is credited also with other significant contributions to our understanding of the morphology of the neuron: 'Freud provided coherent evidence suggesting that the protoplasm consists of a contractile fibrillary network, the present-day cytoskeleton; he was one of the original founders of the fibrillary theory on the structure of the protoplasm. Concerning the biology of the cell nucleus, Freud appears to have been the first author who documented movements of nucleoli in nerve cells, a phenomenon presently referred to as nuclear rotation. In certain instances, Freud's observations antedate later views by more than half a century and are important to our current understanding of cell structure and basic processes of intracellular motility' (Triarhou & Del Cerro, 1987, p. 111).

2 See Freud, (1950 [1895]), pp. 322–3: '*Contact Barriers.* [. . .] We may expect to find that the process of conduction itself will create a differentiation in the protoplasm and consequently an improved conductive capacity for subsequent conduction. Furthermore, the theory of contact barriers can be turned to advantage as follows. A main characteristic of nervous tissue is memory: that is, quite generally, a capacity for being permanently altered by single occurrences – which offers such a striking contrast to the behaviour of a material that permits the passage of a wave movement and thereafter returns to its former condition. A psychological theory deserving any consideration must furnish an explanation of "memory".'

Compare this simple hypothesis to the effect that synapses serve not only conduction but also memory with Sherrington's subsequent (1906) suggestions: 'Such a surface might restrain diffusion, bank up osmotic pressure, restrict the movement of ions, accumulate electric charges, support a double electric layer, alter in shape and surface tension with changes in difference of potential [. . .] or intervene as a membrane between dilute solutions of electrolytes of different concentration or colloidal suspensions with different sign of charge.'

3   Pribram & Gill (1976), p. 67.
4   See Freud (1950 [1895]), pp. 356–7: 'It is in relation to a fellow human being that a human being learns to cognize. Then the perceptual complexes proceeding from this fellow human being will in part be new and non-comparable – his *features*, for instance, in the visual sphere; but other visual perceptions – e.g., those of the movements of his hands – will coincide in the subject with memories of quite similar visual impressions of his own, of his own body, [memories] which are associated with memories of movements experienced by himself. Other perceptions of the object too – if, for instance, he screams – will awaken the memory of his [the subject's] own screaming and at the same time of his own experiences of pain. Thus the complex of the fellow human being falls apart into two components, one of which makes an impression by its constant structure and stays together as a thing, while the other can be *understood* by the activity of memory – that is, can be traced back to information from the [subject's] own body'. Freud (1905a, p. 167 f.) later built upon this passage in a discussion of 'ideational mimetics', where he linked it with the bigger concept of 'empathy'.
5   Gallese (2009).
6   Freud (1933), p. 159.
7   Sacks (1984), p. 164.
8   Chalmers (1995), p. 203. Chalmers explains his use of the term 'function': 'Here "function" is not used in the narrow teleological sense of something that a system is designed to do, but in the broader sense of any causal role in the production of behaviour that a system might perform.'
9   Freud (1940 [1938]), p. 142.
10 By psychophysicists like Gustav Fechner and Wilhelm Wundt.
11 Fotopoulou & Conway (2004), Turnbull, Berry & Evans (2004), Fotopoulou et al. (2007, 2008a,b), Turnbull & Solms (2007), Fotopoulou, Conway & Solms (2007), Fotopoulou (2008, 2009, 2010a,b), Coltheart & Turner (2009), Cole et al. (2014), Besharati, Fotopoulou & Kopelman (2014), Besharati et al. (2014), Turnbull, Fotopoulou & Solms (2014), Kopelman, Bajo & Fotopoulou (2015), Besharati et al. (2016).
12 Solms & Panksepp (2010), Zellner et al. (2011), Yovell et al. (2016).
13 Freud (1940 [1938]), pp. 177–8.
14 Shepherd (1991), p 8.
15 Freud (1940 [1938]), p. 145.
16 Freud (1900), p. 476.
17 Freud (1901), p. 222.
18 Freud (1920), p. 57.
19 Brentano (1924), p. 194.

20 Freud (1940 [1938]), pp. 142–3.
21 Ibid., p. 143.
22 Freud (1950 [1895]), p. 340.
23 Freud (1915a), p. 107; emphasis added.
24 Ostow (1962), pp. 20–1.
25 Carhart-Harris & Friston (2010).
26 Freud (1900), pp. 565–6. (I have slightly amended the official translation here, to make it more comprehensible to the uninitiated.)
27 Kruglanski & Friston (2020).
28 Freud (1900), p. 566; emphasis added.
29 Ibid.
30 Seth (2021b).
31 Freud (1900), p. 567.
32 Hobson & Friston (2012), p. 8.
33 Damasio (2018).
34 Thorndike (1911).
35 Chalmers (1995), pp. 203–4.
36 He was influenced by Claude Bernard, who was a scientific predecessor of Walter Cannon, the biologist who introduced our modern conception of 'homeostasis' in 1929.
37 Freud (1920), p. 57.
38 Letter of December 6, 1896.
39 Freud (1920), p. 25.
40 Bauer (2007).
41 Freud (1935a), p. 28.
42 Zeki (1993), p. 209.
43 Freud (1910), p. 85; emphasis added.
44 Zeki (1993), p. 209.
45 Harlow & Harlow (1962).
46 Zeki (1993), p. 210; emphasis added.

CHAPTER FOUR: The Talking Cure

1 Letter dated February 8, 1934.
2 Ingram (1992).
3 Steinert et al. (2017).
4 Shedler (2010), p. 98.
5 Leuzinger-Bohleber et al. (2019).
6 Cohen (1988, 1992).
7 Smith, Glass & Miller (1980).
8 Robinson, Berman & Neimeyer (1990).

9 Lipsey & Wilson (1993).
10 Turner et al. (2008); Kirsch et al. (2008); Khan, Mar & Brown (2021).
11 Janick et al. (1985).
12 Hidalgo, Tupler & Davidson (2007); Kalwani & Van Buskirk (2017).
13 Leucht et al. (2022).
14 Wykes, Steel, Everitt & Tarrier (2008).
15 Abbass et al. (2006).
16 Here is an operational definition of 'psychoanalytic' therapy: (1) The dialogue between the therapist and the patient is unstructured and open-ended. (This is based on the *free association* technique.) (2) The therapist identifies *recurring patterns* in the patient's associations, and also in their everyday experiences and behaviours. (3) The therapist links these recurring patterns, as they manifest in the patient's current experiences, with *past* experiences – and especially with *childhood* experiences. (4) The therapist 'interprets' these patterns. That is, they attempt to elucidate their *implicit* meaning by rendering *explicit* the predictions which produce the recurring patterns. (5) The therapist draws attention to the patient's *feelings* – and especially to those which the patient tries to avoid and to suppress. (6) The therapist draws attention to the patient's *defensive* manoeuvres in this respect ('can you see that you are doing this in order not to feel that?'). (7) The therapist focuses on the *relationship* between the patient and themselves (this is the narrow definition of 'transference'). (8) The therapist links this relationship with the patient's *other* relationships – present and past – again drawing attention to common patterns (this is the broader definition).
17 Leichsenring & Rabung (2008).
18 De Maat et al. (2009).
19 Leuzinger-Bohleber et al. (2019).
20 Leichsenring et al. (2015).
21 Norcross (2005).
22 Letter dated December 6, 1896.
23 For an accessible review of the physiological processes in question, see Dudai (2000).
24 Bargh & Chartrand (1999), p. 476.
25 I am disregarding 'priming' here (where exposure to a stimulus unconsciously influences the response to a subsequent stimulus).
26 See for example Torres (2019).
27 Bowlby (1969).
28 See for example Gilbert et al. (2009).
29 Freud (1923), p. 15.
30 Here is an operational definition of 'CBT': (1) The dialogue between

the therapist and the patient has a *specific focus*, with the therapist structuring the interaction and introducing the topics. (2) The therapist often functions in a *didactic* or teacher-like manner. (3) The therapist offers explicit *guidance and advice*. (4) The therapist and patient have agreed *treatment goals*. (5) The therapist *explains* the rationale behind the treatment and techniques to the patient. (6) The therapy focuses on the patient's *current* life situation (i.e., not on childhood). (7) The therapy focuses on *cognitive* themes, such as thoughts and belief systems. (8) The therapist *prescribes tasks or activities* ('homework') for the patient to attempt outside of therapy sessions.

This and the previous operational definition (endnote 16) are the *official* versions of what these two types of therapists do, but it doesn't necessarily mean that this is what they actually do. When 'blind' raters are provided with verbatim transcripts of real sessions conducted by CBT practitioners and by psychoanalytic therapists, they frequently have difficulty in identifying which of the two types of therapy is being conducted. Therefore, studies which look beyond the brand names that therapists give to their treatments – by examining what CBT practitioners and psychoanalytic therapists *actually do* (using session videotapes or verbal transcripts) – reveal more about what the 'active ingredients' are that produce the therapeutic effects.

31 Haemodialysis is usually done three times per week. Without it, the serum potassium level rises, and fluid overload becomes fatal within much less than a month, more likely within days, depending on the amount of residual renal function. The work of the kidney, like that of the mind, is continuous. What is also interesting about dialysis vs analysis is that psychoanalysis leads to the internalization of the new function, whereas dialysis doesn't (although renal transplant does).

CHAPTER FIVE: Slips of the Tongue

1 Malcolm (1984), p. 8.
2 He was a second-generation analyst. I was fortunate to befriend two other New York psychoanalysts who knew Freud – the neurologist Else Pappenheim-Frishauf and the psychiatrist Henry Nunberg – but they were children at the time they knew him; they only visited Freud's home with their parents, who were colleagues of his.
3 *The Revised Standard Edition of the Complete Psychological Works of Sigmund Freud*, 24 vols. Lanham, MD: Rowman & Littlefield, 2021.
4 Laplanche (1991), p. 403; Underwood (2004), p. xliv, (2006), n. 8.
5 This accusation is attributable to Laplanche (1992, p. 52), the psychoanalyst

and philosopher who oversaw the translation of Freud's complete psychological works into French.
6. Bettelheim (1983).
7. Freud, 1920, p. 57.
8. Freud (1915b), p. 158.
9. Freud (1900), pp. 565–6.
10. Cobb (2020).
11. Freud (1950 [1895]), p. 319.
12. Solms (2020), p. 7.
13. Pribram & Gill (1976).
14. Ibid.; Pribram (1962, 1965).
15. Kandel (1999), p. 505.
16. Kandel (1998).
17. Friston (2020), p. 57.
18. Freud (1917), p. 158.
19. Freud (1924a), p. 171.
20. Freud (1940 [1938]), p. 179.
21. Freud (1920), p. 38.
22. Letter to Fliess dated December 22, 1897.
23. Freud (1905b), p. 191.
24. All the facts summarized thus far are derived from LeVay (1993), apart from the last one – concerning INAH-3 in male-to-female transgender people – which is derived from Swaab (2008).
25. Freud (1951 [1935]).
26. Freud (1916–17), p. 286; translation very slightly amended.
27. Braun et al. (1997).
28. Panksepp (1998), p. 155.
29. Watt & Panksepp (2009).
30. Tolchinsky et al. (2024).
31. Barrett (2017).
32. E.g., Touroutoglou et al. (2015), p. 1257; Wager et al. (2015), p. 2.
33. See Fourie et al. (2011).

CHAPTER SIX: Defence Mechanisms

1. See Duncan et al. (2016).
2. Freud (1905a), p. 202.
3. Gilgamesh, king of Uruk, believes himself above the limits of ordinary men, but the death of his wildman companion Enkidu disturbs him terribly. Unable to accept the fact of mortality, he embarks on a quest to find the secret of eternal life. He seeks wisdom from the immortal

Utnapishtim, braves distant lands, and even walks along the bottom of the sea in search of a magical plant said to restore youth – only to lose it to a serpent. After all his striving, he returns to Uruk, realizing at last that the grandeur of his city is what will endure. So it did, for something in the region of 3,000 years.
4 Freud (1924b), p. 143.
5 Freud (1914).
6 Freud (1894). To be clear: I don't mean to imply that neurotic, narcissistic or psychotic disorders can be reduced to defences *alone*.
7 *Scientific American*, September 2004, p. 16.
8 Ramachandran (1994).
9 Weinstein & Kahn (1955).
10 Bisiach & Geminiani (1991); McGlynn & Schacter (1989).
11 Ramachandran & Blakeslee (1998).
12 See Turnbull, Fotopoulou & Solms (2014) for a review of this evidence. My colleagues and I have also successfully treated many such patients with psychoanalytic psychotherapy.
13 Freud (1925), pp. 43–4.
14 Freud did not draw the distinction between repression and defence as sharply as I am here. He described repression as being a special case of defence. I don't agree with him, for the reason just stated: repressed predictions are aimed (however badly) at getting rid of needs; defensive predictions are aimed at getting rid of feelings only.
15 Meynert (1884), p. v.
16 At the time of writing this (January, 2025). I randomly checked the list of contents for the latest issue of the *American Journal of Psychiatry*. Here are the titles: 'Spaced Transcranial Direct Current Stimulation for Major Depression', 'Randomized Controlled Trial of the Effects of High-Dose Ondansetron on Clinical Symptoms and Brain Connectivity in Obsessive-Compulsive and Tic Disorders', 'Esketamine Treatment for Depression in Adults: A PRISMA Systematic Review and Meta-Analysis', 'Five-Year Outcomes of a School-Based Personality-Focused Prevention Program on Adolescent Substance Use Disorder: A Cluster Randomized Trial', 'Use of Telemental Health Care by Children and Adolescents in the United States', 'Redefining Ketamine Pharmacology for Antidepressant Action: Synergistic NMDA and Opioid Receptor Interactions?', 'The Impact of Xanomeline and Trospium Chloride on Cognitive Impairment in Acute Schizophrenia: Replication in Pooled Data From Two Phase 3 Trials'.
17 Posse et al. (2018).
18 Mayberg et al. (2005).

19 Mayberg (2006).
20 Emphasis added.
21 See for example Gilbert et al. (2009).
22 Freud (1917).
23 I would be reluctant to generalize this to *all* cases of major depression, such as those diagnosed in Parkinson's disease, frontotemporal dementia, drug detoxification and other abstinence states, Huntington's disease, untreated obstructive sleep apnoea, etc., the final common pathway of all of which can be major depression. This is a big issue with depression: it is more like anaemia than a stand-alone disease. Anaemia from post-partum haemorrhage is very different from pernicious anaemia (due to vitamin B12 deficiency) or iron-deficiency anaemia, or anaemia secondary to a blood malignancy, or anaemia as a medication side effect. These are all 'anaemia' in the strict sense of the word, with a deficit of red blood cells, but their treatment is related to the aetiology. My argument is that in cases of depression which arise from early developmental adversity (i.e., the vast majority of cases, especially in young people), symptomatic treatment is insufficient.
24 Moncrief et al. (2023). An umbrella analysis is a type of research that combines and assesses multiple existing systematic reviews and meta-analyses on a specific topic. It is essentially a 'review of reviews'.
25 https://www.ucl.ac.uk/news/2022/jul/no-evidence-depression-caused-low-serotonin-levels-finds-comprehensive-review
26 Freud (1940 [1938]), p. 164.
27 Yovell et al. (2016) for overall findings; Yovell & Bar (personal communication, 2025) for effect size.
28 Hobson & McCarley (1977), p. 1346.
29 'Brücke carried more weight with me than anyone else in my whole life'; Freud (1926), p. 226.
30 Letter to Hallmann (1842), published in Du Bois-Reymond (1918), p. 108; emphasis added.
31 Shevrin et al. (1992).
32 Freud (1920), p. 57.
33 Freud (1914), p. 68.

CHAPTER SEVEN: The Future of an Illusion

1 Freud (1933), p. 126.
2 Jung (1955), p. 212.
3 Kishimi & Koga (2013).
4 The remark is attributed to Edward Glover (Hansi Kennedy, personal communication, 1996).

5   See King & Steiner (1991).
6   Freud (1915a), pp. 109–10.
7   Freud (1933), p. 71.
8   Lacan (1956), p. 128.
9   Lacan (1960), p. 300.
10 What he actually said is: '*Sa morale relève d'un cynisme supérieur*'. In context, it could also be translated: 'His morality is the domain of a higher cynicism' (Onfray, 2010).
11 Brandell (2010), p. 70.
12 Perlman & Brandell (2014).
13 DeYoung (2003), p. 28.
14 Freud (1915), p. 280.
15 Freud (1940 [1938]), p. 164.

CHAPTER EIGHT: A Cure by Love

1   He moved to a farm that he owned in the former German colony of South West Africa (now Namibia) which was at that time a 'mandate' of South Africa. His children and grandchildren subsequently settled in South Africa proper.
2   Crick (1994), p. 3.
3   Esman (2011).
4   Letter dated July 20, 1938.
5   Deleuze & Guattari (1972), p. 54.
6   Freud (1921), p. 74.
7   Freud (1921), pp. 107–8.
8   Merker (2007); Solms (2021). Other theories of consciousness are, of course, available too.
9   Freud (1920), pp. 37–8.
10 I must clarify that it was not my family who 'took' this particular farm. It was granted to another European settler, in 1690, and bought by my family from his successors in title.
11 Varoufakis (2023).
12 Letter dated December 11, 1921.
13 Letter to Julius Tandler, dated November 29, 1931.
14 Freud (1935b), pp. 273–4.
15 Letter to Israel Cohen, dated June 14, 1938.
16 Freud (1930), p. 89.
17 Freud (1895), p. 272.
18 Letter to Max Halberstadt, dated January 25, 1920.
19 Letter to Carl Jung, dated December 6, 1906.

20 Letter to Albert Einstein, dated March 26, 1929.

EPILOGUE: The Cause

1 Boonzaaier & Mendelow (2023).

References

Abbass, A., Hancock, J., Henderson, J. & Kisely, S. (2006), 'Short-term psychodynamic psychotherapies for common mental disorders', *Cochrane Database of Systematic Reviews*, 4, Article No. CD004687. doi: 10.1002/14651858.CD004687.pub3

Abbass, A., Kisely, S., Town, J., Leichsenring, F., Driessen, E., De Maat, S., Gerber, A., Dekker, J., Rabung, S., Rusalovska, S. & Crowe E. (2014), 'Short-term psychodynamic psychotherapies for common mental disorders' (Review), *Cochrane Database of Systematic Reviews*, 7.

Bacon, M. (2024), 'The therapist who hated me', *Aeon*, April 8, 2024.

Bargh, J. & Chartrand, T. (1999), 'The unbearable automaticity of being', *American Psychologist*, 54: 462–79.

Barrett, L. F. (2017), *How Emotions are Made: The Secret Life of the Brain*. New York: Houghton Mifflin Harcourt.

Bauer, P. (June 2007), 'Recall in infancy: A neurodevelopmental account', *Current Directions in Psychological Science*, 16: 142–6. doi: 10.1111/j.1467-8721.2007.00492.x

Becker, E. (1973), *The Denial of Death*. New York: Simon & Schuster.

Berger, L. (2000), *Freud: Darkness in the Midst of Vision*. New York: Wiley & Sons.

Besharati, S., Forkel, S. J., Kopelman, M., Solms, M., Jenkinson, P. M. & Fotopoulou, A. (2014), 'The affective modulation of motor awareness in anosognosia for hemiplegia: behavioural and lesion evidence', *Cortex*, 61: 127–40.

Besharati, S., Forkel, S., Kopelman, M., Solms, M., Jenkinson, P. & Fotopoulou, A. (2016), 'Mentalizing the body: spatial and social cognition in anosognosia for hemiplegia', *Brain*, 139: 971–85.

Besharati, S., Fotopoulou, A. & Kopelman, M. (2014), 'What is it like to be confabulating?' In A. L. Mishara, A. Kranjec, P. Corlett, P. Fletcher & M. A. Schwartz, eds, *Phenomenological Neuropsychiatry, How Patient Experience Bridges Clinic with Clinical Neuroscience.* New York: Springer.

Bettelheim, B. (1983), *Freud and Man's Soul.* New York: Flamingo.

Bisiach, E. & Geminiani, G. (1991), 'Anosognosia relating to hemiplegia and hemianopia'. In G. Prigatano & D. Schacter, eds, *Awareness of Deficit after Brain Injury: Clinical and theoretical Issues.* New York: Oxford University Press, pp. 25–6.

Boonzaaier, Z. & Mendelow, E. (2023), *The Impact of Early Separation Trauma on Adulthood Depression: Development of the Separation Distress Adversity Scale.* Unpublished thesis: University of Cape Town.

Bowlby, J. (1969), *Attachment.* London: Hogarth Press.

Brandell, J. (2010), *Theory and Practice in Clinical Social Work.* New York: The Free Press.

Braun, A., Balkin, T., Wesenten, N. et al. (1997), 'Regional cerebral blood flow throughout the sleep-wake cycle'. An $H_{2(15)}O$ PET study. *Brain*, 120: 1173–97.

Brentano, F. (1924), *Psychology From an Empirical Standpoint*, 2nd edn. London: Routledge & Kegan Paul (English translation, 1973).

Broca, P. (1861), 'Remarques sur le siège de la faculté du langage articulé, suivies d'une observation d'aphémie (perte de la parole)', *Bulletin de la Société Anatomique de Paris*, 6: 330–57.

Bykhovsky, B. (1926), Метапсихология Фрейда. Monograph: Minsk.

Carhart-Harris, R. & Friston, K. (2010), 'The default-mode, ego-functions and free-energy: a neurobiological account of Freudian ideas', *Brain*, 133: 1265–83.

Chalmers, D. (1995), 'Facing up to the problem of consciousness', *Journal of Consciousness Studies*, 2: 200–19.

Clark, A. (2015), *Surfing Uncertainty: Prediction, Action, and the Embodied Mind.* New York: Oxford University Press.

Cobb, M. (2020), *The Idea of the Brain.* London: Profile Books.

Cohen, J. (1988), *Statistical Power Analysis for the Behavioral Sciences*, 2nd edn. New York: Routledge.

Cohen, J. (1992), 'A power primer', *Psychological Bulletin*, 112: 155.

Cole, M. (1979), 'Introduction: The historical context'. In A. R. Luria, *The Making of Mind*. Cambridge, MA: Harvard University Press, pp. 1–14.

Cole, S., Fotopoulou, A., Oddy, M. & Moulin, C. (2014), 'Implausible future events in a confabulating patient with an anterior communicating artery aneurysm', *Neurocase*, 20: 208–24.

Coltheart, M. & Turner, M. (2009), 'Confabulation and delusion'. In W. Hirstein, ed., *Confabulation: Views from Neuroscience, Psychiatry, Psychology and Philosophy*. New York: Oxford University Press, p. 173.

Crews, F. (1998), *Unauthorized Freud: Doubters Confront a Legend*. New York: Viking.

Crews, F. (2017), *Freud: The Making of an Illusion*. New York: Metropolitan Books/Henry Holt.

Crick, F. (1994), *The Astonishing Hypothesis: The Scientific Search for the Soul*. New York: Charles Scribner's Sons.

Damasio, A. (2018), *The Strange Order of Things: Life, Feeling, and the Making of Cultures*. London: Penguin Random House.

Deleuze, G. & Guattari, F. (1972), *Anti-Oedipus: Capitalism and Schizophrenia*. New York: Viking Press (English translation, 1977).

De Maat, S., De Jonghe, F., Schoevers, R. & Dekker J., 'The effectiveness of long-term psychoanalytic therapy: a systematic review of empirical studies', *Harvard Review of Psychiatry*, 17: 1–23. doi: 10.1080/10673220902742476

Dement, W. & Kleitman, N. (1957), 'The relation of eye movements during sleep to dream activity: an objective method for the study of dreaming', *Journal of Experimental Psychology*, 53: 339–46.

DeYoung, P. (2003), *Relational Psychotherapy: A Primer*. London: Routledge.

Drury, A., Elbert, M. & DeLisi, M. (2019), 'Childhood sexual abuse is significantly associated with subsequent sexual offending:

New evidence among federal correctional clients', *Child Abuse & Neglect*, 95: 104035. https://doi.org/10.1016/j.chiabu.2019.104035

Du Bois-Reymond, E., ed. (1918), *Jugendbriefe von Emil Du Bois-Reymond an Eduard Hallmann, zu seinem hundertsten Geburtstag, dem 7. November 1918*. Berlin: Reimer.

Dudai, Y. (2000), 'The shaky trace', *Nature*, 406: 686–7.

Duncan, A., Malcolm-Smith, S., Ameen, O. & Solms, M. (2016), 'The incidence of euphoria in multiple sclerosis: Artefact of measure', *Multiple Sclerosis International*, 2016: 738425. http://dx.doi.org/10.1155/2016/5738425

Esman, A. (2011), 'Psychoanalysis and Surrealism: André Breton and Sigmund Freud', *Journal of the American Psychoanalytic Association*, 59: 173–81.

Esterson, A. (1993), *Seductive Mirage, An Exploration of the Work of Sigmund Freud*. Chicago: Open Court.

Eysenck, H. (1985), *Decline and Fall of the Freudian Empire*. Harmondsworth: Viking.

Feinstein, J., Adolphs, R., Damasio, A. & Tranel, D. (2011), 'The human amygdala and the induction and experience of fear', *Current Biology*, 21: 34–8. doi: 10.1016/j.cub.2010.11.042

Fourie, M., Rauch, H., Morgan, B., Ellis, G., Jordaan, E. & Thomas, K. (2011), 'Guilt and pride are heartfelt, but not equally so', *Psychophysiology*, 48: 888–99.

Fotopoulou, A. (2008), 'False-selves in neuropsychological rehabilitation: the challenge of confabulation', *Neuropsychological Rehabilitation*, 18: 541–65.

Fotopoulou, A. (2009), 'Disentangling the motivational theories of confabulation'. In W. Histein, ed., *Confabulation: Views from Neurology, Psychiatry, and Philosophy*. New York: Oxford University Press.

Fotopoulou, A. (2010), 'The affective neuropsychology of confabulation and delusion', *Cognitive Neuropsychiatry*, 15: 38–63.

Fotopoulou, A. (2013), 'Beyond the reward principle: consciousness as precision seeking', *Neuropsychoanalysis*, 15: 33–8.

Fotopoulou, A. & Conway, M. (2004), 'Confabulation pleasant and unpleasant', *Neuropsychoanalysis*, 6: 26–33.

Fotopoulou, A., Conway, M., Birchall, D., Griffiths, P. & Tyrer, S. (2007), 'Confabulation: revising the motivational hypothesis', *Neurocase*, 13: 6–15.

Fotopoulou, A., Conway, M. & Solms, M. (2007), 'Confabulation: motivated reality monitoring', *Neuropsychologia*, 45: 2180–90.

Fotopoulou, A., Conway, M., Solms, M., Kopelman, M. & Tyrer, S. (2008a), 'Self-serving confabulation in prose recall', *Neuropsychologia*, 46: 1429–41.

Fotopoulou, A., Conway, M., Tyrer, S., Birchall, D., Griffiths, P. & Solms, M. (2008b), 'Is the content of confabulation positive? An experimental study', *Cortex*, 44: 764–72.

Fotopoulou, A., Solms, M. & Turnbull, O. (2004), 'Wishful reality distortions in confabulation: a case report', *Neuropsychologia*, 42: 727–44.

Frankfurt, H. (2005), *On Bullshit*. Princeton, NJ: Princeton University Press.

Freud, S. (1882), 'Über den Bau der Nervenfasern und Nervenzellen beim Flußkrebs', *Sitzungsberichte der kaiserlichen Akademie der Wissenschaften Wien* (Mathematisch-Naturwissenschaftliche Klasse), Section 3, 85, 9–46.

Freud, S. (1888), 'Gehirn' (Part I: 'Anatomie des Gehirns'). In A. Villaret, *Handwörterbuch der gesamten Medizin*, 1. Stuttgart: Ferdinand Enke, pp. 684–91.

Freud, S. (1891), *Zur Auffassung der Aphasien. Eine kritische Studie*. Vienna: Franz Deuticke.

Freud, S. (1893), 'Some points for a comparison between organic and hysterical motor paralyses', *The Revised Standard Edition of the Complete Psychological Works of Sigmund Freud*, 1: 185–99. Lanham, MD: Rowman & Littlefield.

Freud, S. (1894), 'The neuropsychoses of defence', *The Revised Standard Edition of the Complete Psychological Works of Sigmund Freud*, 3: 41–61. Lanham, MD: Rowman & Littlefield.

Freud, S. (1895), 'Studies on hysteria', *The Revised Standard Edition of the Complete Psychological Works of Sigmund Freud*, 2. Lanham, MD: Rowman & Littlefield.

Freud, S. (1900), 'The interpretation of dreams', *The Revised Standard Edition of the Complete Psychological Works of Sigmund Freud*, 4 & 5. Lanham, MD: Rowman & Littlefield.

Freud, S. (1901), 'The psychopathology of everyday life', *The Revised Standard Edition of the Complete Psychological Works of Sigmund Freud*, 6. Lanham, MD: Rowman & Littlefield.

Freud, S. (1905a), 'Jokes and their relation to the unconscious', *The Revised Standard Edition of the Complete Psychological Works of Sigmund Freud*, 8. Lanham, MD: Rowman & Littlefield.

Freud, S. (1905b), 'Three essays on the theory of sexuality', *The Revised Standard Edition of the Complete Psychological Works of Sigmund Freud*, 7: 112–217. Lanham, MD: Rowman & Littlefield.

Freud, S. (1910), 'Leonardo Da Vinci and a memory of his childhood', *The Revised Standard Edition of the Complete Psychological Works of Sigmund Freud*, 11: 57–123. Lanham, MD: Rowman & Littlefield.

Freud, S. (1912), 'A note on the unconscious in psycho-analysis', *The Revised Standard Edition of the Complete Psychological Works of Sigmund Freud*, 12, 253–61. Lanham, MD: Rowman & Littlefield.

Freud, S. (1914), 'On narcissism: An introduction', *The Revised Standard Edition of the Complete Psychological Works of Sigmund Freud*, 14, 59–89. Lanham, MD: Rowman & Littlefield.

Freud, S. (1915a), 'Drives and their vicissitudes', *The Revised Standard Edition of the Complete Psychological Works of Sigmund Freud*, 14: 99–123. Lanham, MD: Rowman & Littlefield.

Freud, S. (1915b), 'The unconscious', *The Revised Standard Edition of the Complete Psychological Works of Sigmund Freud*, 14: 143–91. Lanham, MD: Rowman & Littlefield.

Freud, S. (1915c), 'Thoughts for the times on war and death', *The Revised Standard Edition of the Complete Psychological Works of Sigmund Freud*, 14: 271–301. Lanham, MD: Rowman & Littlefield.

Freud, S. (1916-17), 'Introductory lectures on psychoanalysis', *The Revised Standard Edition of the Complete Psychological Works of Sigmund Freud*, 15 & 16. Lanham, MD: Rowman & Littlefield.

Freud, S. (1917), 'Mourning and melancholia', *The Revised Standard Edition of the Complete Psychological Works of Sigmund Freud*, 14: 213–31. Lanham, MD: Rowman & Littlefield.

Freud, S. (1920), 'Beyond the pleasure principle', *The Revised Standard Edition of the Complete Psychological Works of Sigmund Freud*, 18: 3–61. Lanham, MD: Rowman & Littlefield.

Freud, S. (1921), 'Group psychology and the analysis of the ego', *The Revised Standard Edition of the Complete Psychological Works of Sigmund Freud*, 18: 65–133. Lanham, MD: Rowman & Littlefield.

Freud, S. (1923), 'The ego and the id', *The Revised Standard Edition of the Complete Psychological Works of Sigmund Freud*, 19: 3–58. Lanham, MD: Rowman & Littlefield.

Freud, S. (1924a), 'The dissolution of the Oedipus complex', *The Revised Standard Edition of the Complete Psychological Works of Sigmund Freud*, 19: 165–73. Lanham, MD: Rowman & Littlefield.

Freud, S. (1924b), 'Neurosis and psychosis', *The Revised Standard Edition of the Complete Psychological Works of Sigmund Freud*, 19: 139–45. Lanham, MD: Rowman & Littlefield.

Freud, S. (1925), 'An autobiographical study', *The Revised Standard Edition of the Complete Psychological Works of Sigmund Freud*, 20: 3–66. Lanham, MD: Rowman & Littlefield.

Freud, S. (1926), 'The question of lay analysis', *The Revised Standard Edition of the Complete Psychological Works of Sigmund Freud*, 20: 159–242. Lanham, MD: Rowman & Littlefield.

Freud, S. (1927), 'The future of an illusion', *The Revised Standard Edition of the Complete Psychological Works of Sigmund Freud*, 21: 3–52. Lanham, MD: Rowman & Littlefield.

Freud, S. (1930), 'Civilization and its discontents', *The Revised Standard Edition of the Complete Psychological Works of Sigmund Freud*, 21: 55–131. Lanham, MD: Rowman & Littlefield.

Freud, S. (1933), 'New introductory lectures on psychoanalysis', *The Revised Standard Edition of the Complete Psychological Works of Sigmund Freud*, 22: 3–160. Lanham, MD: Rowman & Littlefield.

Freud, S. (1935a), 'An autobiographical study', *The Revised Standard Edition of the Complete Psychological Works of Sigmund Freud*, 20: 3–66. Lanham, MD: Rowman & Littlefield.

Freud, S. (1935b), 'Letter to the Society of B'Nai Brith, Vienna', *The Revised Standard Edition of the Complete Psychological Works of Sigmund Freud*, 22: 273–4. Lanham, MD: Rowman & Littlefield.

Freud, S. (1940 [1938]), 'An outline of psychoanalysis', *The Revised Standard Edition of the Complete Psychological Works of Sigmund Freud*, 23: 127–87. Lanham, MD: Rowman & Littlefield.

Freud, S. (1950 [1895]), 'Project for a scientific psychology', *The Revised Standard Edition of the Complete Psychological Works of Sigmund Freud*, 1: 309–421. Lanham, MD: Rowman & Littlefield.

Freud, S. (1951 [1935]), 'Letter on homosexuality', *The Revised Standard Edition of the Complete Psychological Works of Sigmund Freud*, 22: 270–71. Lanham, MD: Rowman & Littlefield.

Freud, S. (2012 [1885–87]), 'Kritische Einleitung in die Nervenpathologie'. In K. Günther, G. Fichtner & A. Hirschmüller, eds, *Luzifer-Amor*, 25: 33–82.

Freund, K., Watson, R. & Dickey, R. (1990), 'Does sexual abuse in childhood cause pedophilia: an exploratory study', *Archives of Sexual Behavior*, 19: 557–68. doi: 10.1007/BF01542465

Friston, K. (2020), 'The importance of being precise', *Neuropsychoanalysis*, 22: 57–61.

Gallese, V. (2009), 'Mirror neurons, embodied simulation, and the neural basis of social identification', *Psychoanalytic Dialogues*, 19: 519–36. https://doi.org/10.1080/10481880903231910

Gilbert, R., Widom, C., Browne, K., et al. (2009), 'Burden and consequences of child maltreatment in high-income countries', *Lancet*, 373: 68–81. doi: 10.1016/S0140-6736(08)61706-7

Grinstein, A. (1956–75), *The Index of Psychoanalytical Writings*, 14 vols. New York: International Universities Press.

Harlow, H. & Harlow, M. (1962), 'Social deprivation in monkeys', *Scientific American*, 207: 136–46. http://dx.doi.org/10.1038/scientificamerican1162-136

Hidalgo, R., Tupler, L. & Davidson, J. R. (2007), 'An effect-size analysis of pharmacologic treatments for generalized anxiety disorder', *Journal of Psychopharmacology*, 21: 864–72. doi: 10.1177/0269881107076996

Hobson, J. A. (1988), *The Dreaming Brain*. New York: Basic Books.

Hobson, J. A. (2011), *Dream Life: An Experimental Memoir*. Cambridge, MA: MIT Press.

Hobson, J. A. & McCarley, R. (1977), 'The brain as a dream state generator: an activation-synthesis hypothesis of the dream process', *American Journal of Psychiatry*, 134: 1335–48.

Hobson, J. A. & Friston, K. (2012), 'Waking and dreaming consciousness: neurobiological and functional considerations', *Progress in Neurobiology*, 98: 82–98.

Hohwy, J. (2013), *The Predictive Mind*. New York: Oxford University Press.

Ingram, D. (1992), Review of Strenger's 'Between Hermeneutics and Science: An Essay on the Epistemology of Psychoanalysis', 1991. *American Journal of Psychoanalysis*, 52: 297–8.

Jackson, M. & Solms, M. (2013), 'Separation distress in obsessive-compulsive disorder', *Neuropsychoanalysis*, 15: 117–25.

Janick et al. (1985), 'Efficacy of ECT: A meta-analysis', *American Journal of Psychiatry*, 142: 297–302.

Joravsky, D. (1974), 'A great Soviet psychologist', *New York Review of Books*, 16 May, 21: 22–5.

Jouvet, M. (1965), 'Paradoxical sleep: a study of its nature and mechanisms', *Progress in Brain Research*, 18: 20–62.

Jung, C. G. (1955), 'Aion: Researches into the Phenomenology of the Self', *The Collected Works of C. G. Jung*, 9 (Part 2). Princeton: Princeton University Press.

Kalwani, R. & Van Buskirk, J. (2017), 'Are benzodiazepines effective for treatment of generalized anxiety disorder?', *Evidence-Based Practice*, 20: E8–E9. doi: 10.1097/01.EBP.0000541748.97949.e2

Kandel, E. (1998), 'A new intellectual framework for psychiatry', *American Journal of Psychiatry*, 155: 457–69.

Kandel, E. (1999), 'Biology and the future of psychoanalysis: a new intellectual framework for psychiatry revisited', *American Journal of Psychiatry*, 156: 505–24.

Kant, I. (1784), 'Idea for a universal history with a cosmopolitan purpose'. In H. S. Reiss, ed., *Kant. Cambridge Texts in the History of Political Thought*. Cambridge: Cambridge University Press. pp. 41–53.

Khan, A., Mar, K. & Brown, W. (2021), 'Consistently modest antidepressant effects in clinical trials: The role of regulatory requirements', *Psychopharmacology Bulletin*, 51: 79–108.

King, P. & Steiner, R. (1991), *The Freud-Klein Controversies 1941–45*. London: Routledge.

Kirsch, I., Deacon, B., Huedo-Medina, T., Scoboria, A., Moore, T. & Johnson, B. (2008), 'Initial severity and antidepressant benefits: a meta-analysis of data submitted to the Food and Drug Administration', *PLoS Medicine*, 5: e45. doi: 10.1371/journal.pmed.0050045

Kishimi, I. & Koga, F. (2013), *The Courage to be Disliked*. New York: Simon & Schuster.

Kleist, K. (1934), *Gehirnpathologie*. Leipzig: Barth.

Kline, P. (1972), *Fact and Fantasy in Freudian Theory*. London: Methuen.

Kozulin, A. (1984), *Psychology in Utopia*. Cambridge, MA: MIT Press.

Kruglanski, A., Jasko, K. & Friston, K. (2020), 'All Thinking is "Wishful" Thinking', *Trends in Cognitive Sciences* 24: 413–24.

Lacan, J. (1956), 'The Freudian thing, or the meaning of the return to Freud in psychoanalysis', *Écrits: A Selection*. London: Tavistock, pp. 114–45 (English translation, 1977).

Lacan, J. (1960), 'The subversion of the subject and the dialectic of desire in the Freudian unconscious', *Écrits: A Selection*. London: Tavistock, pp. 292–325 (English translation, 1977).

Laplanche, J. (1991), 'Specificity of terminological problems in the translation of Freud', *International Review of Psychoanalysis*, 18: 401.

Laplanche, J. (1992), *Seduction, Translation, Drives*. London: ICA.

Lebzeltern, G. (1983), 'Freud und das Kokain', *Wiener Klinische Wochenschrift*, 95: 765–9.

Leichsenring, F. & Leibing, E. (2003), 'The effectiveness of psychodynamic therapy and cognitive behavior therapy in the treatment of personality disorders: a meta-analysis', *American Journal of Psychiatry*, 160: 1223–32. doi: 10.1176/appi.ajp.160.7.1223

Leichsenring, F., Rabung, S. & Leibing, E. (2004), 'The efficacy of short-term psychodynamic psychotherapy in specific psychiatric disorders: a meta-analysis', *Archives of General Psychiatry*, 61: 1208–16. doi: 10.1001/archpsyc.61.12.1208

Leichsenring, F. & Rabung, S. (2008), 'Effectiveness of long-term psychodynamic psychotherapy: a meta-analysis', *Journal of the American Medical Association*, 300: 1551–65. doi: 10.1001/jama.300.13.1551

Leichsenring, F., Luyten, P., Hilsenroth, M., Abbass, A., Barber, J., Keefe, J., Leweke, F., Rabung, S. & Steinert, C. (2015), 'Psychodynamic therapy meets evidence-based medicine: a systematic review using updated criteria', *Lancet Psychiatry*, 2: 648–60. doi: 10.1016/S2215-0366(15)00155-8

Leucht, S., Chaimani, A., Krause, M., Schneider-Thoma, J., Wang, D., Dong, S., Samara, M., Peter, N., Huhn, M., Priller, J. & Davis, J. (2022), 'The response of subgroups of patients with schizophrenia to different antipsychotic drugs: a systematic review and meta-analysis', *Lancet Psychiatry*, 9: 884–93. doi: 10.1016/S2215-0366(22)00304-2

Leuzinger-Bohleber, M., Hautzinger, M., Fiedler, G., Keller, W., Bahrke, U., Kallenbach, L., Kaufhold, J., Ernst, M., Negele, A., Schoett, M., Küchenhoff, H., Günther, F., Rüger, B., & Beutel, M. (2019), 'Outcome of psychoanalytic and cognitive-behavioural long-term therapy with chronically depressed patients: A controlled trial with preferential and randomized allocation', *The Canadian Journal of Psychiatry*, 64: 47–58. https://doi.org/10.1177/0706743718780340

LeVay, S. (1993), *The Sexual Brain*. Cambridge, MA: MIT Press.

Lipsey, M. & Wilson, D. (1993), 'The efficacy of psychological, educational, and behavioral treatment. Confirmation from meta-analysis', *American Psychologist*, 48: 1181–209. doi: 10.1037//0003-066x.48.12.1181

Lobner, H. & Levitin, V. (1978), 'A short account of Freudism: Notes on the history of psychoanalysis in the USSR', *Sigmund Freud Haus Bulletin*, 2: 5–30.

Loftus, E. (1994), *The Myth of Repressed Memory: False Memories and Allegations of Sexual Abuse*. New York: St. Martin's Press.

Luria, A. R. (1932a), *The Nature of Human Conflicts*. New York: Liveright.

Luria, A. R. (1932b), 'Psychological expedition to Central Asia', *Journal of Genetic Psychology*, 40: 241–2.

Luria, A. R. (1940), 'психоанализа', большая советская энциклопедия, 13: 248–9.

Luria, A. R. (1947), *Traumatic Aphasia*. The Hague: Mouton (English translation, 1970).

Luria, A. R. (1948), *Restoration of Functions after Brain Injury*. Oxford: Pergamon Press (English translation, 1963).

Luria, A. R. (1962), *Higher Cortical Functions in Man*. New York: Basic Books (English translation, 1966; second edn, 1980).

Luria, A. R. (1963), *Human Brain and Psychological Processes*. New York: Harper & Row (English translation, 1966).

Luria, A. R. (1968), *The Mind of a Mnemonist*. New York: Basic Books.

Luria, A. R. (1976), *Basic Problems of Neurolinguistics*. The Hague: Mouton.

Luria, A. R. (1976), *The Neuropsychology of Memory*. New York: Wiley & Sons.

Luria, A. R. (1972), *The Man with a Shattered World*. New York: Basic Books.

Luria, A. R. (1973), *The Working Brain*. London: Penguin.

Luria, A. R. (1979), *The Making of Mind*. Cambridge, MA: Harvard University Press.

Luria, A. R. & Vygotsky, L. (1930), *Ape, Primitive Man and Child*. New York: Harvester (English translation, 1932).

Luria, A. R. & Majovski, L. V. (1977), 'Basic approaches used in American and Soviet clinical neuropsychology', *American Psychologist*, 32: 959–68. https://doi.org/10.1037/0003-066X.32.11.959

Malcolm, J. (1984), *In the Freud Archives*. New York: Alfred A. Knopf.

Masson, J. M. (1984), *The Assault on Truth: Freud's Suppression of the Seduction Theory*. New York: Farrar Straus Giroux.

Mayberg, H., Lozano, A., Voon, V., McNeely, H., Seminowicz, D., Hamani, C., et al. (2005), 'Deep brain stimulation for treatment-resistant depression', *Neuron*, 45: 651–60. doi: 10.1016/j.neuron.2005.02.014

Mayberg (2006), 'Deep brain stimulation for treatment-resistant depression: An expert interview', *Medscape*, January 5, 2006.

McCarley, R. & Hobson, J. A. (1977), 'The neurobiological origins of psychoanalytic dream theory', *American Journal of Psychiatry*, 134: 1211–21.

McGlynn, S. M. & Schacter, D. L. (1989), 'Unawareness of deficits in neuropsychological syndromes', *Journal of Clinical and Experimental Neuropsychology*, 11: 143–205.

Mecacci, L. (1988), 'Review of A. R. Luria, "The Mind of a Mnemonist" and "The Man With a Shattered World"', *Journal of the History of the Behavioral Sciences*, 24: 268–70.

Merker, B. (2007), 'Consciousness without cerebral cortex: A challenge for neuroscience and medicine', *Behavioral & Brain Sciences*, 30: 63–8.

Meynert, T. (1884), *Psychiatry: A Clinical Treatise on Diseases of the Fore-Brain, Based Upon a Study of its Structure, Functions and Nutrition*. New York: G. P. Punam's & Sons (English translation, 1885).

Miller, M. (1998), *Freud and the Bolsheviks*. New Haven, CT: Yale University Press.

Moncrieff, J., Cooper, R., Stockmann, T. et al. (2023), 'The serotonin theory of depression: A systematic umbrella review of the evidence', *Molecular Psychiatry*, 28: 3243–56. https://doi.org/10.1038/s41380-022-01661-0

Nagel, T. (1974), 'What is it like to be a bat?' *The Philosophical Review*, 83: 435–50.

Norcross, J. C. (2005), 'The psychotherapist's own psychotherapy:

Educating and developing psychologists', *American Psychologist*, 60: 840–50.

Obholzer, K. (1982), *The Wolf Man. Sixty Years Later*. New York: Continuum.

Olds, J. & Milner, P. (1954), 'Positive reinforcement produced by electrical stimulation of septal area and other regions of rat brain', *Journal of Comparative and Physiological Psychology*, 47: 419–27. doi: 10.1037/h0058775

Onfray, M. (2010), 'En finir avec Freud', *Philosophie*, 36: 10–15.

Ostow, M. (1992), *Drugs in Psychoanalysis and Psychotherapy*. New York: Basic Books.

Panksepp, J. (1998), *Affective Neuroscience*. New York: Oxford University Press.

Pappenheim, E. (1990), 'Psychoanalysis in the Soviet Union', *American Psychoanalyst*, 24: 4–5.

Parr, T., Pezzulo, G. & Friston, K. (2022), *Active Inference*. Cambridge, MA: MIT Press.

Perlman, F. & Brandell, J. (2014), 'Psychoanalytic theory'. In J. Brandell, ed., *Essentials of Clinical Social Work*. New York: Sage Publications, pp. 42–83. https://doi.org/10.4135/9781483398266.n3

Popper, K. (1934), *The Logic of Scientific Discovery*. New York: Basic Books (English translation, 1959).

Popper, K. (1963), *Conjectures and Refutations*. New York: Basic Books.

Popper, K. (1974), 'Replies to my critics'. In P. A. Schilpp, ed., *The Philosophy of Karl Popper*, 2. La Salle, IL: Open Court.

Posse, P., Choi, K., Holtzheimer, P., Crowell, A., Garlow, S., Rajendra, J., et al. (2018), 'A connectomic approach for subcallosal cingulate deep brain stimulation surgery: Prospective targeting in treatment-resistant depression', *Molecular Psychiatry*, 23: 843–9. doi: 10.1038/mp.2017.59

Pribram, K. (1962), 'The neuropsychology of Sigmund Freud'. In A. J. Bacharach, ed., *Experimental Foundations of Clinical Psychology*. New York: Basic Books, pp. 442–68.

Pribram, K. (1965), 'Freud's "Project": An open, biologically based model for psychoanalysis'. In N. Greenfield & W. Lewis, eds,

Psychoanalysis and Current Biological Thought. Madison: University of Wisconsin Press, pp. 81–92.

Pribram, K. & Gill, M. (1976), *Freud's 'Project' Re-Assessed. Preface to Contemporary Cognitive Theory and Neuropsychology*. New York: Basic Books.

Pribram, K. & Luria, A. R. (1973), *Psychophysiology of the Frontal Lobes*. New York: Academic Press.

Ramachandran, V. S. (1994), 'Phantom limbs, neglect syndromes, repressed memories, and Freudian psychology', *International Review of Neurobiology*, 37: 291–333; discussion 369–72. doi: 10.1016/s0074-7742(08)60254-8

Ramachandran, V. S. & Blakeslee, S. (1998), *Phantoms in the Brain*. New York: William Morrow.

Robinson, L., Berman, J., Neimeyer, R. (1990), 'Psychotherapy for the treatment of depression: a comprehensive review of controlled outcome research', *Psychological Bulletin*, 108: 30–49. doi: 10.1037/0033-2909.108.1.30

Sacks, O. (1984), *A Leg to Stand On*. New York: Simon & Schuster.

Seth, A. (2021a), *Being You*. London: Faber.

Seth, A. (2021b), 'How the brain accomplishes perception'. https://www.joinexpeditions.com/exps/872

Shannon, C. (1948), 'A mathematical theory of communication', *Bell System Technical Journal*, 27: 379–423.

Shedler, J. (2010), 'The efficacy of psychodynamic psychotherapy', *American Psychologist*, 65: 98–109.

Shem, S. (1978), *The House of God*. New York: Richard Marek Publishers.

Shepherd, G. (1991), *Foundations of the Neuron Doctrine*. Oxford: Oxford University Press.

Sherrington, C. (1906), *The Integrative Action of the Nervous System*. New Haven: Yale University Press.

Shevrin, H., Williams, W., Marshall, R. & Brakel, L. (1992), 'Event-related potential indicators of the dynamic unconscious', *Consciousness and Cognition*, 1: 340–66.

Shorter, E. (1997), *A History of Psychiatry: From Era of the Asylum to the Age of Prozac*. Hoboken, NJ: John Wiley & Sons.

Skinner, B. F. (1953), *Science and Human Behavior.* London: Macmillan.

Smith, M. L., Glass, G. V., & Miller, T. I. (1980), *The Benefits of Psychotherapy.* Baltimore, MD: Johns Hopkins University Press.

Solms, M. (1997), *The Neuropsychology of Dreams: A Clinico-Anatomical Study.* Mahwah, NJ: Lawrence Erlbaum Associates.

Solms M. (2000), 'Dreaming and REM sleep are controlled by different brain mechanisms', *Behavioral & Brain Sciences,* 23: 843–50.

Solms, M. (2020), 'New project for a scientific psychology: General scheme', *Neuropsychoanalysis,* 22: 5–35. doi: 10.1080/15294145.2020.1833361

Solms, M. (2021), *The Hidden Spring: A Journey to the Source of Consciousness.* London: Profile Books.

Solms, M. (2022), 'Revision of Freud's theory of the biological origin of the Oedipus complex', *Psychoanalytic Quarterly,* 90: 555–81. doi.org/10.1080/00332828.2021.1984153

Solms, M. & Panksepp, J. (2010), 'Why depression feels bad'. In E. Perry, D. Collerton, F. LeBeau & H. Ashton, eds, *New Horizons in the Neuroscience of Consciousness.* Amsterdam: John Benjamins, pp. 169–79.

Steinert, C., Munder, T., Rabung, S., Hoyer, J. & Leichsenring, F. (2017), 'Psychodynamic therapy: As efficacious as other empirically supported treatments? A meta-analysis testing equivalence of outcomes', *American Journal of Psychiatry,* 174: 943–53. doi: 10.1176/appi.ajp.2017.17010057

Sulloway, F. (1979), *Freud, Biologist of the Mind.* New York: Basic Books.

Swaab, D. (2008), 'Sexual orientation and its basis in brain structure and function', *Proceedings of the National Academy of Sciences,* 105: 10273–4. https://doi.org/10.1073/pnas.0805542105

Swales, P. (1982), 'Freud, Minna Bernays, and the Conquest of Rome: New Light on the Origins of Psychoanalysis', *The New American Review,* 1: 1–23.

Thorndike, E. (1911), *Animal Intelligence.* New York: Macmillan.

Thornton, E. (1983), *The Freudian Fallacy: Freud and Cocaine*. London: Blond & Briggs.

Timpanaro, S. (1974), *The Freudian Slip: Psychoanalysis and Textual Criticism*. New York: Verso.

Tolchinsky, A., Ellis, G., Levin, M., Kaňková, Š. & Burgdorf, J. (2024), 'Disgust as a primary emotional system and its clinical relevance', *Frontiers of Psychology*, 15. doi: 10.3389/fpsyg.2024.1454774

Tolman E. (1948), 'Cognitive maps in rats and men', *Psychological Review*, 55: 189–208.

Torres, N. (2019), 'Testing a neuro-evolutionary theory of social bonds and addiction: Methadone associated with lower attachment anxiety, comfort with closeness, and proximity maintenance', *Frontiers in Psychiatry*, 10. doi: 10.3389/fpsyt.2019.00602

Touroutoglou, A., Lindquist, K., Dickerson, B. & Barrett, L. F. (2015), 'Intrinsic connectivity in the human brain does not reveal networks for "basic" emotions', *Social, Cognitive and Affective Neuroscience*, 10: 1257–65. doi: 10.1093/scan/nsv013

Triarhou, L. & Del Cerro, M. (1987), 'The histologist Sigmund Freud and the biology of intracellular motility', *Biology of the Cell*, 61: 111–14. doi: 10.1111/j.1768-322x.1987.tb00576.x

Turnbull, O. Berry, H. & Evans, C. (2004), 'A positive emotional bias in confabulatory false beliefs about place', *Brain and Cognition*, 55: 490–94.

Turnbull, O., Fotopoulou, A. & Solms, M. (2014), 'Anosognosia as motivated unawareness: the "defence" hypothesis revisited', *Cortex*, 61: 18–29.

Turnbull, O., Jenkins, S. & Rowley, M. (2004), 'The pleasantness of false beliefs: an emotion-based account of confabulation', *Neuropsychoanalysis*, 6: 5–16.

Turnbull, O. & Solms, M. (2007), 'Awareness, desire, and false beliefs', *Cortex*, 43: 1083–90.

Turner, E., Matthews, A., Linardatos, E., Tell, R. & Rosenthal, R. (2008), 'Selective publication of antidepressant trials and its influence on apparent efficacy', *New England Journal of Medicine*, 358: 252–60. doi: 10.1056/NEJMsa065779

Underwood, J. (2004). In S. Freud, *Mass Psychology and Other Writings*. London: Penguin.

Underwood, J. (2006). In S. Freud, *Interpreting Dreams*. London: Penguin.

Valkanova, Y. (2016), 'The Psychoanalytic Kindergarten Project in Soviet Russia 1921–1930', *SCRSS Digest*, 13: 12–15.

Van der Veer, R. & Valsiner, J. (1991), *Understanding Vygotsky*. Oxford: Blackwell.

Varoufakis, Y. (2023), *Technofeudalism: What Killed Capitalism*. London: Bodley Head.

Wager, T., Kang, J., Johnson, T., Nichols, T., Satpute, A. & Barrett, L. F. (2015), 'A Bayesian model of category-specific emotional brain responses', *PLoS Computational Biology*, 11: e1004066. doi: 10.1371/journal.pcbi.1004066

Watt, D. & Panksepp, J. (2009), 'Depression: An evolutionarily conserved mechanism to terminate separation distress? A review of aminergic, peptidergic, and neural network perspectives', *Neuropsychoanalysis*, 11: 7–51. https://doi.org/10.1080/15294145.2009.10773593

Webster, R. (2005), *Why Freud was Wrong: Sin, Science and Psychoanalysis*. London: Orwell Press.

Weinstein, E. A., & Kahn, R. L. (1955), *Denial of Illness: Symbolic and physiological aspects*. Springfield, IL: Charles C. Thomas. https://doi.org/10.1037/11516-000

Wykes, T., Steel, C., Everitt, B., Tarrier, N. (2008), 'Cognitive behavior therapy for schizophrenia: effect sizes, clinical models, and methodological rigor', *Schizophrenia Bulletin*, 34: 523–37. doi: 10.1093/schbul/sbm114

Yovell, Y., Bar, G., Mashiah, M. et al. (2016), 'Ultra-low-dose buprenorphine as a time-limited treatment for severe suicidal ideation: a randomized controlled trial', *American Journal of Psychiatry*, 173: 491–8.

Zeki, S. (1993), *A Vision of the Brain*. Oxford: Blackwell.

Zellner, M., Watt, D., Solms, M. & Panksepp, J. (2011), 'Affective neuroscientific and neuropsychoanalytic approaches to two intractable psychiatric problems: why depression feels so bad and what addicts really want', *Neuroscience and Biobehavioral Reviews*, 35: 2000–2008.

Acknowledgements

I would like to thank my colleagues – psychiatrists and psychoanalysts – Andrea Clarici (Trieste), Gyuri Fodor (Vienna), Tennyson Lee (London), Steven Yeates (Sydney), Yoram Yovell (Jerusalem) and Michelle van den Engh (Vancouver) for their helpful comments on a near-final draft of this book. Of course, my gratitude does not imply that they carry any responsibility for the opinions I have expressed.

I would like also to thank my darling poet and artist Eliza Kentridge for keeping me passably literate – not to mention deeply happy.

As for my editor, Ed Lake, it is difficult to convey how indebted I am to him for transforming my plodding scientific writing into a more-than-readable book. Like many people, I was under the erroneous impression that editors like him don't exist anymore.

Finally, I would like to thank my remarkable agent, Caroline Dawnay, and acknowledge that it was her idea that I should write a book about Freud, following the publication of my *Revised Standard Edition* of his psychological works.

Index

Abbass, Allan 282, 289, 299
acetylcholine, *see* neuromodulators
addiction 11, 113, 118, 144, 168, 186, 197, 198, 228
ADHD 110, 181, 185, 194
Adler, Alfred 208
affect, *see* feelings
Aichhorn, August 131
amygdala 42–3, 117
anaclisis 78, 132, 212
anal sexuality, *see* sexuality
anorexia nervosa 168, 197
anosognosia 11, 70, 164, 174–7, 197, 228
apartheid 248–51, 256
Aristotle 15
artificial intelligence 78, 228
attachment (*see also* drives: CARE, PANIC/GRIEF) 92, 94, 118–19, 135, 143–4, 148, 153, 156, 160, 181, 197, 254, 257
attention deficit disorder, *see* ADHD
Auden, Wystan Hugh 10, 277
autism 181, 187, 195–7
automatization, *see* memory

Bacon, Michael 210, 289
Bargh, John 282, 289
Barrett, Lisa Feldman 157–8, 219, 284, 289, 305, 306

Barthes, Roland 143
basal ganglia 117, 204
basic emotions, *see* drives
Beck, Aaron 103
Beck, Ludwig 234
Becker, Ernest 237, 289
behaviourism 35, 67, 86–7, 89, 211, 220
benzodiazapines, *see* psychiatric medications
Bergson, Henri 78
Bernard, Claude 281
Bernays, Edward 143
Bernays, Martha, *see* Freud, Martha
Berridge, Kent 48, 152
Besharati, Sahba 280, 289–90
Bettelheim, Bruno 133, 214, 284, 290
biogenetic law 36, 269
Bion, Wilfred 220
bipolar disorder 186
bisexuality, *see* sexuality
Bisiach, Edoardo 285, 290
Bleuler, Eugen 207
body/mind relationship, *see* mind/body relationship
Boonzaaier, Zürika 288, 290
Bowlby, John 94–5, 119, 211–13, 282, 290
brainstem (*see also* cerebellum; midbrain; pons) 46–7, 49, 91
Braun, Allen 284, 290

Breger, Louis 38
Brenner, Charles 8, 227
Brentano, Franz 75, 281, 290
Breton, André 239–40
Broca, Paul 17, 277, 290
Brücke, Ernst 199, 286
Buddha 152
Butler, Judith 240
Bykhovsky, Bernard 23, 25, 290

Canaris, Wilhelm 233, 234
Cannon, Walter 281
Cajal, Santiago Ramón y 64, 71
CARE, *see* drives
Carhart-Harris, Robin 281, 290
cases
    Johan T 166–8, 171, 173, 198
    Lord N 203–6, 229
    Mabel D 99–102, 125
    Paulina Z 43, 62
    SM 43, 223
    Teddy P 1–5, 6, 7, 13, 187, 194, 263–76
    thirty-something woman 122–3, 126
    Thomas W 164–6, 171, 173, 177, 178, 183, 187
    Wolf Man, the 37, 130
cathexis 132–3, 135
causes vs symptoms 5, 7, 13, 14, 113, 191–5, 197–8, 260
CBT 103–4, 106, 111–13, 124, 127, 189
    defined 282–3
cerebellum 117, 133
Chalmers, David 67–8, 87, 280, 281, 290
Charcot, Jean Martin 60–1, 165, 183–8, 191, 195–6, 201
Chartrand, Tanya 282, 289
childhood, importance of (*see also* critical periods; infantile amnesia) 13, 25–6, 27, 92–5, 96, 127, 282
choice 86, 128, 242–3
Clark, Andy 82, 290
Clarici, Andrea 308
Cobb, Matthew 64, 66, 72, 136, 284, 290
cocaine 10, 37, 113, 144–5, 194
cognitive behavioural therapy, *see* CBT
Cole, Michael 27, 278, 291
colonialism 24, 246–51, 256
coma 91, 236, 257
confabulatory amnesia, *see* Korsakoff syndrome
conflict, mental 25, 28, 149, 159–60
consciousness (*see also* uncertainty) 11, 68–9, 75, 85–6, 87, 89, 90–1, 96, 114–16, 120, 135, 170, 180, 228, 242–5
consolidation, *see* memory
Copernicus 238
corpus callosum 133, 146
countertransference, *see* transference/countertransference
Crews, Frederick 38–9, 291
Crick, Francis 238, 287, 291
critical periods 91–5, 146, 161–2

Da Vinci, Leonardo 93, 149
Dalí, Salvador 240
Damasio, Antonio 86, 227, 242, 281, 291, 292
Darwin, Charles 39, 75, 238
Dawnay, Caroline 308
DBS 6, 188–9
De la Porte, Jean-Pierre 49, 51, 215
De Maat, Saskia 282, 289, 291
De Saussure, Ferdinand 213–14

INDEX

death anxiety, *see* mortality
death drive, *see* drives
declarative memory, *see* memory
deep brain stimulation, *see* DBS
defences (*see also* repression)
   164–202, 248, 282
  denial 171, 174–7
  disavowal 173
  introjection 173, 176
  projection 101, 168, 171, 173, 176
  projective identification 65
  rationalization 174, 251
  reaction formation 174
  sublimation 34, 63, 173
delusion 173, 181, 221
Deleuze, Gilles 240, 287, 291
depression 4, 5, 6, 11, 70, 107–8,
   109–12, 120, 139, 140, 143, 152–3,
   181, 185, 186, 187–93, 196, 197,
   199, 228, 263–5, 286
  animal models of 6–7
  co-morbidity with panic disorder
   4, 196
  serotonin deficiency hypothesis
   6, 191–3
depth psychology 61, 74, 89, 120, 202
Derrida, Jacques 217
Descartes, René 16, 68, 137, 221
Diagnostic and Statistical Manual
   of Mental Disorders, *see* DSM
Diogenes the Cynic 216
Disgust 157
dopamine, *see* neuromodulators
Dostoevsky, Fyodor 22
dreams (*see also* hallucination) 4,
   11, 27, 33, 53, 62, 69, 84, 85–6,
   91, 198–9
  give expression to wishes 9, 22–3,
   33, 43–4, 46, 48, 91, 152–3, 228
  in neurological patients 43–5,
   47–8
  in Urbach-Wiethe disease 43–4
  latent vs manifest 22–3, 33, 116
  neuropsychology of 44–8
  relation to REM sleep 45–7
drives (*see also* homeostasis;
   instincts; libido; sexuality), 74,
   77–82, 86, 88, 150–63, 213, 218,
   222, 224, 228, 256–7
  CARE 153–4, 157, 160, 190, 231,
   257–62, 275–6
  death 78, 139–40, 244–5
  FEAR 43, 97–8, 155, 156, 157, 159,
   160, 180, 222–6, 254, 257, 261
  LUST 145, 148, 154–5, 157, 160, 161,
   254, 257, 261
  PANIC/GRIEF 119–20, 144, 145,
   148, 151, 153, 154, 157, 159, 160,
   181, 194, 196, 224, 254, 261, 271
  PLAY 120–2, 139, 154–5, 157, 160,
   161, 203, 254, 257, 261
  RAGE 15, 155, 157, 159, 160, 181,
   224, 236, 254–5, 261
  SEEKING 42, 48, 145, 148, 152–3,
   157, 160, 181, 194, 261
DSM 150, 161, 185–7, 189–90, 196
Du Bois-Reymond, Emil 199, 286,
   292
Duncan, Amy 284, 292

ECT 6, 110, 189, 197
Einstein, Albert 9, 10, 262, 288
Eissler, Kurt 129–33, 227, 283
Eissler, Ruth 130
Ekman, Paul 157
electroconvulsive therapy, *see* ECT
Ellis, Havelock 174
embodied cognition (*see also*
   enactment) 65, 96
emotional memory, *see* memory

emotions, *see* drives; feelings
empathy 155, 228, 254, 280
enactment 54, 55, 116, 122–6, 134, 169, 219
epigenetics 95, 197, 228
episodic memory, *see* memory
Esterson, Allen 39, 292
Eysenck, Hans 38, 292

Fairbairn, Ronald 211
falsifiability/falsification 32–6, 38, 46, 48, 67, 141, 176, 200, 221–2
Fanon, Frantz 240
FEAR, *see* drives
Fechner, Gustav 280
feelings (*see also* subjectivity) 12, 50, 70, 81, 86–8, 96, 120–2, 135, 147–8, 151, 171, 172, 178–81, 210, 218–19, 222, 242, 248, 282
Feyerabend, Paul 35–6
fixation 92, 121, 145, 161
Fliess, Wilhelm 88–9, 114, 141, 162, 284
Fodor, Gyuri 308
forced swim test 6–7
Fonagy, Peter 227
Fotopoulou, Aikaterini 280, 285, 289–90, 291, 292–3, 305
Fourie, Melike 284, 292
Frankfurt, Harry 32, 278, 293
free association 33, 53, 62, 74, 228, 282
free energy 79–82, 137
free will, *see* choice
Freud, Anna 52–3, 209–13
Freud, Martha (*née* Bernays) 129
Freud, Sigmund (*see also* psychoanalysis)
   Archives at the Library of Congress 37, 129, 131

   as a Jew 26, 207, 253–4
   as a microscopist 56–7, 64, 71
   as a neurologist 9, 49–50, 65, 69
   as a neuropsychologist 40, 49, 65
   as a neuroscientist 9, 10, 49, 56–61, 64–5, 69, 96, 129, 133, 279
   as a scientist 10, 14, 30, 34, 40, 67, 133–4, 137, 139, 199–202, 221–2, 225, 252
   busts and portraits of 8, 9
   clichéd images of 9, 113
   criticisms of 9–10, 23, 25, 31, 33–9, 63, 149, 208, 239
   influence upon Luria 22, 29–30, 61, 65–6
   theories consistent with modern neuroscience 12, 40, 64–96, 113–14, 117, 118, 138, 148–9, 200–1
   theories important for the future of psychiatry and neuroscience 40–1, 66–96, 138, 174–7, 215, 226
   translation of 11, 40, 56, 129, 132–9, 214–15, 308
Freud, Sophie 258
Friston, Karl 78, 80–1, 83, 85, 137–8, 227, 281, 284, 290, 296, 297, 298, 302
functional neurological disorder 49–50, 60, 140, 174, 176, 182, 184–5, 228
functionalism 18, 20, 58–9, 72–4, 76, 96, 135, 198–9

gain from illness 171, 266
Galen 16, 32
Galileo 31
Gall, Franz Joseph 16
Gallese, Vittorio 65, 280, 296

INDEX

Geschwind, Norman 19
Glover, Edward 286
glucocorticoids, *see* neuromodulators
Goethe, Johann Wolfgang 131, 146, 244
Golgi, Camillo 71
Green, André 8, 227
Grinstein, Alexander 27, 296
Groddeck, Georg 202
group psychology 240–1
Guattari, Félix 240, 287, 291
guilt 159, 235–6, 248, 256

habituation, *see* psychiatric medications
Haeckel, Ernst (*see also* biogenetic law) 36
hallucination 33, 45, 83–6, 93, 136, 181
Hansen, Georg 234
Hardenberg, Carl-Hans 234
Harlow, Harry 94–5, 281, 296
HDRF 6, 95
Hebb, Donald 19, 65
Hécean, Henry 19
Hegel, Wilhelm Friedrich 213
Heidegger, Martin 213
Helmholtz, Hermann 81, 138
heterosexuality, *see* sexuality
Himmler, Heinrich 234–5
Hippocrates 16
Hitler, Adolph 62, 232–6, 240
Hobbes, Thomas 78
Hobson, J. Allan 45–8, 85–6, 136–7, 198, 278, 281, 286, 297, 301
Hohwy, Jakob 82, 297
homeostasis 86–7, 119, 136, 140, 155–6, 179, 281
homosexuality, *see* sexuality

Hope for Depression Research Foundation, *see* HDRF
Hume, David 16
hypothalamic-pituitary-adrenal axis 95
hypothalamus 147, 284
hysteria, *see* functional neurological disorder

ICD 185
infantile amnesia 91–2, 119, 228
information (*see also* free energy; predictive processing) 73, 81, 96, 137, 228
instincts (*see also* drives) 82, 119–20, 151, 154, 155–8, 162
International Classification of Diseases, *see* ICD
interpretation, *see* transference/countertransference

Jackson, John Hughlings 29, 51
Jackson, Michelle 196, 297
Jones, Ernest 252–3
Joravsky, David 27, 278, 297
Jouvet, Michel 47, 297
Jung, Carl 206–8, 220, 286, 288, 297

Kaiser Wilhelm II 232
Kandel, Eric 137, 227, 284, 297–8
Kant, Immanuel 135, 279, 298
Kaplan, Karen 226
Kennedy, Hansi 286
Kentridge, Eliza 308
ketamine, *see* psychiatric medications
King, Pearl 287, 298
Klein, Melanie (*see also* psychoanalysts: Kleinian) 131, 209–13
Kline, Paul 36, 38

Kölliker, Rudolph 71
Kolmar, Gertrud 235
Kopelman, Michael 280, 289–90, 293
Korsakoff syndrome 11, 70, 228
Kozulin, Alex 26, 278, 298

Lacan, Jacques 213–17, 287, 298
Lakatos, Imre 35–6
Lake, Ed 308
Lamarck, Jean Baptiste 36
language, brain mechanisms of 16–17, 18–19, 21, 29, 49, 58, 65–6
Laplanche, Jean 132, 283–4, 298–9
Laufer, Eglé 100–2, 168
learning from experience 82–3, 86–7, 115–16, 151
Lebzeltern, Gustav 113
Le Doux, Joseph 227
Le Vay, Simon 284, 299
Lee, Tennyson 308
Leichsenring, Falk 282, 289, 298–9, 304
Lenin, Vladimir 23, 26
Leonardo, *see* Da Vinci, Leonardo
Leuzinger-Bohleber, Marianne 281, 282, 299
libido (*see also* drives; narcissism; sexuality) 4, 77–8, 79, 121–2, 142–5, 161, 212, 257
Lipschitz, Robert 51–2
localizationism 18–20, 60
    dynamic localization of functional systems 19–20, 57–60, 65–6, 69–70
Locke, John 16
Loftus, Elizabeth 37–8, 300
long-term memory, *see* memory
love 135, 143, 153, 160, 190, 224, 239, 261

a cure by 259, 261
thy neighbour as thyself 252–6, 261
Luria, Aleksandr Romanovich, 137, 158, 277–8, 300–1, 303
    as father of neuropsychology 19, 40
    as psychoanalyst 22–30, 40
    chapters missing from The Working Brain 24, 29, 69–70, 228
    dynamic localization of functional systems 19–20, 45, 65–6, 69–70
    major neuropsychological works of 21
    syndrome analysis 20, 61, 69–70, 196
LUST, *see* drives

Mabel D, *see* cases
major depressive disorder, *see* depression
Malcolm, Janet 129–30, 283, 301
mania 181
Marcuse, Herbert 240
Marx, Karl 10, 23, 26, 35
Masson, Jeffrey 37, 129, 141, 301
Mayberg, Helen 188, 227, 285–6, 301
Meaney, Michael 95
Mecacci, Luciano 29, 278, 301
medial forebrain bundle, *see* mesocortical/mesolimbic dopamine system
memory (*see also* infantile amnesia; learning from experience; predictive processing; repression) 13, 55, 64–5, 70, 73, 74, 83, 84, 89–92, 114–20, 279
    automatization 117–19, 123, 127,

135, 148, 151–2, 178, 216
consolidation 89–90, 115, 117–18, 127, 151
declarative (*see also* preconscious) 90, 91–2, 114–17, 119, 123, 135
emotional 114, 118
episodic 114, 117, 119, 127
false (*see also* Korsakoff syndrome) 37–8, 141
long-term 89–92, 114–15
multiple systems 88–91, 96, 114–20
nondeclarative (*see also* unconscious, the) 114, 116–20, 124, 126, 127, 148, 151, 156, 172
priming 282
procedural 114, 118
reconsolidation 89–91, 115, 119, 282
semantic 114, 117–19, 127
short-term (*see also* consciousness) 89–90, 114, 115
Mendelow, Ella 288, 290
Merker, Bjorn 287, 301
mesocortical/mesolimbic dopamine system (*see also* neuromodulators) 48, 152
metapsychology 61, 74, 87, 135, 158
methylphenidate, *see* psychiatric medications
Meynert, Theodor 57, 60, 181–4, 191, 194, 199, 201–2, 220, 260, 301
Michelangelo 149
midbrain 115, 133, 243
Miller, Jacques-Alain 216
mind/body relationship (*see also* functionalism; localizationism) 15–21, 49–51, 59–60, 68, 72–4, 75–6, 182, 202, 238

mirror neurons 65, 280
Moncrieff, Joanna 192, 286, 301
mortality 55, 206, 229, 237–9
multiple memory systems, *see* memory
multiple sclerosis 164–5, 173, 183
myalgic encephalomyelitis 140

Näcke, Paul 174
Nagel, Thomas 277, 301
Nansen, Fridtjof 71
Nazis (*see* also Hitler, Adolph) 10, 35, 54, 130, 232–6
narcissism 10, 174, 238–9, 240, 244–5
Nersessian, Edward 227
neuromodulators 91, 115, 121, 179, 187, 193, 198
  acetylcholine 46, 48
  glucocorticoids 95, 185
  dopamine 48, 144–5, 148, 152–3, 192–3
  mu opioids 144, 148, 197
  noradrenaline 192
  oestrogen 95, 144, 146, 153
  oxytocin 144, 146, 153
  prolactin 153
  progesterone 153
  serotonin (*see also* depression; psychiatric medications) 6, 191–3
  substance P 155
  testosterone 144, 146
  vasopressin 144, 146
neuropsychology, 226
  birth of 17, 19
  clinico-anatomical method 44, 183
  double dissociation of function 47

neuropsychology—*contd.*
  excludes the psyche 67–8, 226
  of dreams, *see* dreams
  prehistory of 15–18
neuropsychoanalysis 68–70, 226–9
Newton, Isaac 39
Nietzsche, Friedrich 10, 78
nondeclarative memory, *see*
  memory
Norcross, John 282, 301–2
Nunberg, Henry 283

Obholzer, Karin 37, 302
obsessive-compulsive disorder, *see*
  OCD
OCD 141, 185, 186, 196, 197, 228
Oedipus complex 9, 34, 145, 160,
  206, 247
oestrogen, *see* neuromodulators
opiates, *see* psychiatric medications
Ostow, Mortimer 79, 137, 226–7, 281,
  302

panic disorder 11, 140, 156, 181, 185,
  196, 228
  co-morbidity with depression 4,
  196
PANIC/GRIEF, *see* drives
Panksepp, Jaak 48, 68, 119, 151–3,
  157, 161, 197, 227, 280, 284, 302,
  304, 306
Pappenheim, Else 278, 283, 302
paranoia 15, 159, 204, 215
parapraxis 9, 33, 36, 61
Parkinson's disease 11, 286
Parr, Thomas 78
Pauli, Wolfgang 32, 278
Paulina Z, *see* cases
penis envy 9, 139, 145
perceptual identity, *see*
  hallucination
perception 15, 24, 44, 70, 72, 73, 76,
  81, 83–5, 96, 114, 136
periaqueductal grey 243
personality disorders 111, 112, 122–3,
  150, 181, 186
perversion 161, 186
Pezzulo, Giovanni 78
Pfeffer, Arnold 226–7
Pfister, Oskar 241
phantasy 123, 141, 212
phobias 61, 156, 180, 197
Planck, Max 8
Plato 149
PLAY, *see* drives
pleasure/unpleasure 78, 86, 121,
  139–40, 142, 144, 148, 150
pons 46–7, 133
post-traumatic stress disorder, *see*
  PTSD
Popper, Karl (*see also* falsifiability/
  falsification) 31–6, 40, 48, 67,
  141, 222, 278, 279, 302
preconscious 89, 114–15, 123, 135
predictive processing 80, 82–6,
  90–1, 96, 115, 122–7, 180, 196–7,
  224
Pribram, Karl 19, 21, 65, 137, 280,
  284, 302–3
pride 235
primary and secondary processes
  85, 117, 135
procedural memory, *see* memory
projection, *see* defences
projective identification, *see*
  defences
psychedelics, *see* psychiatric
  medications
psychiatric medications (*see also*
  causes vs symptoms; ECT;

INDEX

TMS; DBS; vagus nerve stimulation)
antipsychotics 110, 193–4
benzodiazapines 4, 110, 156, 194, 222–3
effectiveness of 104, 110, 260
habituation to 5
ketamine 5
methylphenidate 110
opiates 4, 118, 144, 194, 197
psychedelics 5–6
side effects of 4–5, 186, 193–4, 202, 260
SSRIs 4, 6, 110, 189, 191
psychiatry (*see also* psychiatric medications)
biological 8, 174, 202
preference for physiological treatments 8, 13, 182–3, 191–4, 201, 202, 260–1, 285
psychical reality 62, 67, 70, 201, 219, 243
psychoanalysis (*see also* anaclisis; attachment; cathexis; childhood, importance of; conflict, mental; defences; depth psychology; drives; enactment; fixation; free association; Freud, Sigmund; functionalism; gain from illness; group psychology; infantile amnesia; love; memory; metapsychology; narcissism; neuropsychoanalysis; Oedipus complex; parapraxis; penis envy; phantasy; pleasure/unpleasure; preconscious; primary and secondary processes; psychical reality; psychoanalysts; psychotherapy; reality testing; reconstruction; regression; repression; return of the repressed; sleeper effect; subjectivity; superego, the; therapeutic alliance; transference/countertransference; trauma; unconscious, the; wish fulfilment; working through)
all talking therapies are derived from 9, 103
effectiveness of (*see also* sleeper effect) 13, 102–5, 110–13, 217, 229
loss of influence of 8–9, 23–30, 33, 35, 62, 104
mechanism of cure in 7, 103, 122–8, 222–4, 229
of children 9, 209–10
renaissance of 9, 277
schools of (*see also* psychoanalysts) 206–22
psychoanalysts (*see also* psychoanalysis)
Jungian 207–8
Kleinian 131, 181, 209–13, 220
Lacanian 213–17, 220
once fashionable 7–8
overly confident of their theories 8, 209–10, 220
relational 217–20
turn away from Freud 10, 103
psychopharmacology, *see* psychiatric medications
psychotherapy (*see also* CBT; psychoanalysis) 188–9, 195
almost all forms derived from psychoanalysis 9, 103, 109
as reparenting 260
effectiveness of 13, 109–10
psychoanalytic, defined 282

PTSD 156, 180, 185, 187, 197, 223
Putnam, Hilary 73

RAGE, *see* drives
rapid eye movement, *see* dreams
Ramachandran, Vilaynur 174–7, 227, 285, 303
Rank, Otto 208
reality testing 84–5, 135, 222
reconsolidation, *see* memory
reconstruction 93–4, 131
Reich, Wilhelm 78, 208
Reil, Johann 182
REM sleep, *see* dreams
regression 84
repression (*see also* defences; return of the repressed) 26, 33, 34, 37, 54–5, 63, 103, 122–4, 140, 174, 177–8, 200–1, 228, 240, 244, 285
return of the repressed 172, 256
right cerebral hemisphere 175–6
Rizzolatti, Giacomo 65
Robertson, James 212
Rosenzweig, Saul 34, 103

Sacks, Oliver 28, 67, 69, 226–7, 280, 303
schizophrenia 110, 181, 182, 185, 186, 195–6, 214
Schleswig-Holstein, Adelheid 234
Schopenhauer, Arthur 78
Schulenburg, Friedrich-Werner 234
Schwartz, James 227
secondary process, *see* primary and secondary processes
SEEKING, *see* drives
Segal, Hannah 8
selective serotonin reupdate inhibitors, *see* psychiatric medications

semantic memory, *see* memory
separation distress, *see* drives, PANIC/GRIEF
serotonin, *see* neuromodulators
Seth, Anil 82, 85, 281, 303
sexual trauma (*see* trauma)
sexuality (*see also* libido; narcissism) 77–8, 87–8, 140–51, 162, 239
    anal 10, 121, 143, 161
    bisexuality 145, 149
    genital 121, 143, 161
    heterosexuality 145, 149
    homosexuality 145, 147, 149–50, 252–3
    infantile 141–2, 161
    oral 121, 142–3, 161, 268–9
    phallic 121–2, 143, 145, 161
Shakespeare, William 130
shame 235–6, 248
Shannon, Claude 81, 137, 303
Shedler, Jonathan 104–5, 281, 303
Shem, Samuel 249, 303
Shepherd, Gordon 64, 71, 280, 303
Sherrington, Charles 64–5, 279–80, 303
Shevrin, Howard 200, 227, 286, 303
short-term memory, *see* memory
side effects, *see* psychiatric medications
Skinner, Burrhus Frederic 35, 278, 304
slavery 246–51, 256
sleeper effect 13–14, 113, 195
SM, *see* cases
Solms, Elsie Sylvia v
Solms, Friedrich III 232–6, 245
Solms, Friedrich IV 234–6
Solms, Friedrich V 245
Solms, Johann Adam 246

Solms, Lee 50–1
Solms, Mark ii, 38, 82, 145, 160, 174, 196, 278, 280, 284, 287, 289, 292, 293, 297, 304, 305, 306
Solms, Rudolf 245
Solms, Wilhelm 130
somatic symptom disorders (*see also* functional neurological disorder) 111, 186
somatoparaphrenia 176
Sontag, Susan 143
Soviet Union 10, 21, 24, 26, 27, 233
Spurzheim, Johann 16
SSRIs, *see* psychiatric medications
Stalin, Joseph 10, 24–9, 240
Stalin, Vasily 26
Stauffenberg, Claus 234
Steiner, Riccardo 287, 298
Steinert, Christiane 281, 299, 304
Stekel, Wilhelm 208
Stengel, Erwin 56
Stern, Daniel 210
Stockard, Charles 92
Strachey, James 133–5, 137, 159, 162–3
Strenger, Carlo 103
subjectivity (*see also* feelings) 12, 31, 32–3, 45, 47, 66–71, 72, 75, 81, 86, 96, 103, 135, 141, 148, 149, 176, 200–1, 211, 219–20, 223–4, 238, 242
sublimation, *see* defences
Sulloway, Frank 36, 56, 278, 304
superego, the 25, 28, 133, 159–60
superior colliculi 243
Surrealism 213, 239–40
Swales Peter 36–7, 304
symptoms vs causes, *see* causes vs symptoms
syndromes (*see also* Luria, Aleksandr Romanovich: syndrome analysis) 20, 61, 121, 183, 185, 195–6

Teddy P, *see* Cases
Teuber, Hans-Lukas 19
therapeutic alliance 169
Thorndike, Edward 281, 304
Thornton, Elizabeth 37, 304–5
Timpanaro, Sebastiano 36, 305
TMS 6, 197
Tolchinsky, Alexey 284, 305
Tolman, Edward 89, 305
Tourette's syndrome 28
transcranial magnetic stimulation, *see* TMS
transference/countertransference (*see also* enactment) 53, 55, 65, 99, 100, 124–6, 169, 177, 213, 219, 221, 250, 282
   interpretation 125–7
trauma (*see also* PTSD) 10, 43, 180–1, 186
   sexual 37–8, 101–2, 140–1
Tresckow, Henning 234
Trotsky, Leon 25–6
Trott, Adam 234
Turnbull, Oliver 280, 285, 293, 305

uncertainty 90–1, 115–16, 180
unconscious, the (*see also* automatization) 22–3, 31, 38, 71, 75–7, 96, 114, 116, 127, 134–5, 139, 148, 200–1, 208, 210, 215–16, 240, 282
Underwood, Jim 132, 283, 306
unpleasure, *see* pleasure/unpleasure
Urbach-Wiethe disease 42–4, 223

vagus nerve stimulation 6, 197
Valkanova, Yordanka 26, 278, 306

Van den Engh, Michelle 308
Varoufakis, Yanis 287, 306
vascular dementia 204
voluntary action (*see also* choice) 83–4, 243
Vygotsky, Lev 22, 26, 27, 300

Watt, Douglas 284, 306
Webster, Richard 38, 306
Weinstein, Edwin 175, 285, 306
Willis, Thomas 16
wish fulfilment (*see also* dreams) 9, 82–6, 123, 136, 176
Witzleben, Erich 234
Wolf Man, the, *see* cases

working through 126–8
Wundt, Wilhelm 280

Yeates, Steven 308
Yorke, Clifford 52–5, 98, 124, 125, 173, 227
Yovell, Yoram 197, 280, 286, 306, 308

Zangwill, Oliver 19
Zeki, Semir 93–4, 281, 306
Zellner, Margaret 280, 306
Žižek, Slavoj 240
Zweig, Stefan 240

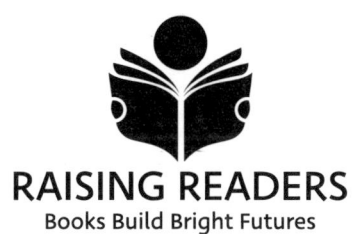

RAISING READERS
Books Build Bright Futures

Dear Reader,

We'd love your attention for one more page to tell you about the crisis in children's reading, and what we can all do.

Studies have shown that reading for fun is the **single biggest predictor of a child's future life chances** – more than family circumstance, parents' educational background or income. It improves academic results, mental health, wealth, communication skills, ambition and happiness.[1]

The number of children reading for fun is in rapid decline. Young people have a lot of competition for their time. In 2024, 1 in 10 children and young people in the UK aged 5 to 18 did not own a single book at home.[2]

Hachette works extensively with schools, libraries and literacy charities, but here are some ways we can all raise more readers:

- Reading to children for just 10 minutes a day makes a difference
- Don't give up if children aren't regular readers – there will be books for them!
- Visit bookshops and libraries to get recommendations
- Encourage them to listen to audiobooks
- Support school libraries
- Give books as gifts

There's a lot more information about how to encourage children to read on our website: **www.RaisingReaders.co.uk**

Thank you for reading.

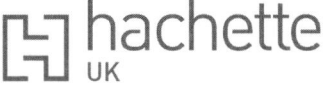

---

[1] National Literacy Trust, Book Ownership in 2024, November 2024
https://nlt.cdn.ngo/media/documents/Book_ownership_in_2024

[2] OECD. 2021. 21st-century readers: developing literacy skills in a digital world. Paris, France: OECD Publishing.
https://www.oecd.org/en/publications/21st-century-readers_a83d84cb-en.html